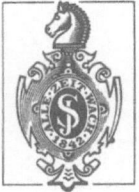

Klaus Poeck

Diagnostic Decisions in Neurology

With a Foreword by
Robert J. Joynt

Springer-Verlag
Berlin Heidelberg New York Tokyo

Professor Dr. med. KLAUS POECK

Head, Department of Neurology
Rheinisch-Westfälische Technische Hochschule
Pauwelsstraße
5100 Aachen, FRG

ISBN-13:978-3-642-70695-0   e-ISBN-13: 978-3-642-70693-6
DOI: 10.1007/978-3-642-70693-6

Library of Congress Cataloging in Publication Data. Poeck, Klaus. Diagnostic decisions in neurology. Includes index. 1. Nervous system — Diseases — Diagnosis. 2. Neurologic examination. 3. Symptomatology. I. Title. [DNLM: 1. Nervous System Diseases — diagnosis.   WL 141 P743d] RC348.P64   1985   616.8′075   85-18801

Typesetting, printing and bookbinding: Universitätsdruckerei H. Stürtz AG, D-8700 Würzburg.
2125/3130-543210

Foreword

Throughout the course of history it has always been noted that any ideas about brain function depended upon the highest technological model of the day. Hence, in the Greek or Roman era the ventricular system was singled out because of the development of hydraulics. Early in this century we drew the analogy between telephone circuits and the brain. Now it is popular to characterize neural function as that of a sophisticated computer. Indeed, in many ways it may be. But, as yet, the prepared human brain will likely prevail in the sorting out of information necessary for a proper diagnosis. In this manual, Dr. POECK has provided the ground work for such preparation.

We all admire the clever diagnostician, and usually ascribe the skill to great intuition. Not so! It is the clinician who has seen many patients, and has compiled a menu of choices. Dr. POECK is such a clinician, and he has provided us with his menu of choices. Use of these lists will likely aid the student or resident physician in coming to a proper diagnosis but, more importantly, will help train his or her mind to think in a logical and systematic way.

ROBERT J. JOYNT, M.D., Ph.D.
Professor of Neurology and Dean
School of Medicine and Dentistry
University of Rochester

Preface

The introduction of new technology for the localization of alterations in the peripheral or central nervous system has provided invaluable assistance to the diagnostician. It cannot be denied, however, that blind faith in, and uncritical application of, these ancillary methods have also produced many false-positive findings. The latter have resulted in unnecessary further and quite often invasive technical examinations, in superfluous operative and medical treatment, and in psychological trauma to the patient.

One should not, it is true, attempt to turn back the clock and practise medicine, in particular make diagnoses, intuitively, as though it were an art beyond rational control. However, it is important not to lose sight of the fact that the signs and symptoms with which the patient presents are a combination of "objective" and "subjective" elements. Every medical practitioner who has been active in the profession long enough will know that not only are objective signs grouped in characteristic patterns, but subjective complaints (i.e., symptoms) are likewise presented in rather stereotypical ways. Disease states have their histories, and one has to learn these as carefully as the signs found in physical and ancillary examinations. If an additional laboratory finding provided, for example, by neuroimaging of the spinal cord or recording of sensory evoked potentials, does not correspond to the history the patient has reported, then we should question the significance of the laboratory findings.

It follows that the art of the diagnostician consists to a large extent of listening attentively to the patient's history. This is not passive listening; during every stage of the interview one has to build up hypotheses which are tentatively confirmed or rejected as careful questioning or, rather, soliciting of details proceeds. At the end of history taking the field of diagnostic possibilities should be narrowed to such a degree that the physical examination, however important, is very unlikely to yield any surprise findings. Ancillary examinations can then be selected for clearly defined purposes.

This book is based on 30 years of work in the field of neurology. For more than half of this time, I have been giving a course on neurologic differential diagnosis. I have attempted to write the kind of hand book that reflects a pragmatic approach to diagnosis. The introductory chapter will give some indication as to how to use this little book.

I have learned a lot from my patients, and have taken every chance to profit from valuable discussions with my closest collaborators W. HACKE, M. HASSEL, E.B. RINGELSTEIN, and H. ZEUMER.

Aachen, Summer 1985 KLAUS POECK

How to Use This Book

This book is intended to provide assistance at the bedside or in the consultation room. To this end, I have refrained from detailed discussion of anatomical or physiological aspects. Likewise, there will be very few, if any, considerations of treatment, as these are given in the available textbooks of neurology.

The chapters do not correspond to anatomical regions or parts of the nervous system, since in many instances we do not know at the beginning of the diagnostic procedure where to locate the disease process. Nor are the chapters centered on disease entities, because these will be recognized only at the end, not at the beginning of our diagnostic considerations. The chapter headings highlight prototypical situations reported by patients, or patterns of signs and symptoms. Consequently, the chapters are in alphabetical order.

At the beginning of each chapter the principal diagnoses that have to be taken into consideration are listed. This list, with numbered items corresponding to the sequence of items in the text, will immediately give the reader an idea of the challenge he has to meet in a given situation. For each diagnostic possibility the pros and cons are then discussed, and the potential contribution of ancillary examinations is evaluated. Extensive cross-referencing is intended to facilitate comparison with similar situations or patterns of findings.

It is hoped that on the basis of the suggestions given in this book the reader will more easily be able to recognize the condition with which the patient is afflicted.

Contents

XII

1 Abnormal Posture of the Head

In the conditions discussed in this chapter the head is either turned or tilted to one side, or both. The description is not comprehensive, in that abnormal posture as observed in comatose or poorly reactive patients following extensive damage to the cerebral hemispheres and/or brain stem is not analyzed. The pathophysiological mechanism underlying the abnormal posture in these patients, who are mostly to be found in the intensive care unit, is inadequately known, especially since many of these patients harbor more than one CNS lesion.

1.1 Unilateral Paralysis of Extraocular Muscles

The most frequent cause is unilateral paralysis of one of the extraocular muscles.

1.1.1 Trochlear Nerve Palsy

It may be difficult to detect the vertical divergence of the eyes in trochlear nerve palsy. Frequently, the patients do not give a very clear description of diplopia on downward gaze, e.g., when walking downstairs. Most of them, however, keep their head turned and tilted toward the nonaffected side in order to compensate for the paralyzed inward rotating function of the superior oblique muscle. If the head and gaze are held straight, one may notice a slight elevation of the affected eye, which increases when the eye is abducted, because in this position the superior oblique muscle should move the eye downward. The vertical divergence becomes most evident when the head is tilted toward the affected side, because now the action of the superior rectus muscle is not balanced at all by the superior oblique muscle (Bielschowskys sign).

1

1.1.2 Abducent Nerve Palsy

Many but not all patients with abducent nerve palsy try to avoid double vision by turning the head toward the affected side, which compensates the paralyzed lateral version of the eye. In the primary position there may be a convergent squint, which increases when the eyes are moved toward the affected side, as does double vision.

1.2 Complete Homonymous Hemianopia

Damage to the visual pathways after they have partially crossed in the optic chiasm causes complete homonymous hemianopia. The patients are "blind" in the visual field contralateral to the side of the lesion. Some of them instinctively compensate for the loss of one hemifield by keeping the head turned toward the blind side. There is no head tilt. Ocular movements are normal unless hemianopia is accompanied by either paralysis of the horizontal gaze or contralateral neglect. In both instances the patient is unable or at least quite reluctant to move the eyes toward the hemianopic field. It may be very difficult, if not impossible, to differentiate gaze paralysis from neglect. The hemianopia is demonstrated at the bedside by the so called confrontation method: the patient is asked to fixate the examiner, who keeps his arms outstretched to both sides at the level of his head. The task for the patient is to distinguish whether the examiner's fingers move on one or the other side, or simultaneously on both sides.

1.3 Paralysis of Horizontal Gaze

Damage either to the frontal or parietal and occipital lobes of the cerebral hemisphere, or to the brain stem causes paralysis of horizontal gaze. As a rule of thumb it may be stated that the cerebral oculomotor centers "push" the gaze to the contralateral side. Consequently, damage to the hemispheres or to the pathways down to the brain stem leads to conjugate deviation of the eyes toward the affected side. If there is hemiparesis, ocular deviation is toward the nonparalyzed limbs. In contrast to hemianopia, the patients do not compensate for the gaze paralysis by turning the head toward the paralyzed side, i.e., away from the lesion. On the contrary, quite often not only the eyes but also the head is turned toward the side of the lesion. As a rule, hemispheric gaze paralysis is transient.

In brain stem lesions at the pontine level there is paralysis of horizontal gaze toward the side of the lesion. In severe cases, there is deviation both of the eyes and of the head toward the paralyzed limbs, and this deviation lasts much longer than in hemispheric affections.

1.4 Ocular Tilt

A rare triad consisting of ipsilateral tilting of the head, conjugate torsion of the eyes, and slow deviation, where the ipsilateral eye is deviated downward, constitutes ocular tilt. The syndrome indicates an ipsilateral brain stem lesion at the level of the midbrain tegmentum. In rare instances, the syndrome is brought about by a lesion in the ipsilateral utriculus, the part of the peripheral vestibular organ (labyrinth) which is involved in the regulation of body posture.

1.5 Posterior Fossa Tumor

There may be tilting of the head toward the side of the lesion, which is not accompanied by overt oculomotor dysfunction or by any visual field defect, in the case of tumor of the posterior fossa. In the old literature the phenomenon was called "vestibular tilt." Headache, neck stiffness, and papilledema are quite suggestive of the diagnosis, which is easily confirmed by neuroimaging.

1.6 Paralysis of the Accessory Nerve

Both the sternomastoid muscle and the upper part of the trapezius muscle are innervated by the accessory nerve. Since the action of each of the sternomastoid muscles rotates the head toward the opposite side, paralysis of one of them interferes with the physiological balance between the two. The result is a position in which the head is slightly turned toward the side of the paralyzed muscle, and the chin is somewhat elevated in the same direction.

1.7 Retroflexion of the Head in Ocular Myopathy

Any kind of ocular myopathy that weakens elevation of the eyelids and/or the eyes will lead to compensatory retroflexion of the head.

Various diagnoses must be considered. Myasthenia gravis is characterized by weakness upon exercise (see also Chap. 40), which is alleviated by intravenous injection of substances inhibiting acetylcholinesterase. Dysthyrotic ocular myopathy is not necessarily recognized by pathologic laboratory findings. Quite regularly, however, neuroimaging of the orbit demonstrates swelling of the extraocular muscles, which provides the correct diagnosis. Slowly progressing weakness of the extraocular muscles is seen in a group of disease processes, the nosologic status of which is still a matter of debate. In part, these are variants of muscular dystrophy; in part, the weakness is neurogenic; and there

3

are combinations with dysfunction in other subsystems of the central and peripheral nervous system, which are summarized under the term "ophthalmoplegia plus."

1.8 Benign Ocular Torticollis

A rare type of ocular torticollis is seen in infancy. These children present with turning and tilting of the head to one side, to the effect that both eyes are kept relatively still at the medial and lateral angle of the orbit. This is to avoid oscillating movements of the eyes that grossly interfere with normal vision. In addition, there is an irregular tremor of the head. Signs and symptoms are not present during sleep, and the triad subsides after a period of months or years. Etiology is unknown.

2 Acute Blindness

2.1 Bilateral Infarction of Posterior Cerebral Artery (Top of the Basilar Embolus)

By far the most frequent cause of acute blindness is bilateral ischemia evolving toward infarction in the territory of the posterior cerebral artery. Of course, this requires occlusion of the top of the basilar artery where, as a rule, the posterior cerebral arteries branch off. Usually this is due to an embolus originating somewhere proximally, probably in one of the vertebral arteries. This is an emergency, because if the diagnosis is made within roughly 5 h of origin, intra-arterial thrombolytic therapy has a fair chance of success.

Embolism at the top of the basilar artery does not usually occur without warning. All of our patients have had transient premonitory symptoms pointing to brain stem dysfunction for several days prior to the event, sometimes even longer. These include unilateral or bilateral paresthesias of the upper limbs, locomotor ataxia, unilateral weakness, slurred speech, and hemianopia or diplopia. The diagnostic problems of acute basilar artery occlusion are discussed in detail in Chap. 31. Here we are concerned with the particular problem of acute cortical blindness. Localization in the occipital lobe is suggested by the absence or severe impairment of vision in the presence of normal pupillary reactions to light. Some patients exhibit Anton's syndrome, i.e., anosognosia – unawareness of blindness. The pattern of behavior is very characteristic. The patient will show an orienting reaction to acoustic stimuli, which betrays the absence of vision. He will not complain of blindness, which he may even categorically deny. Yet, when walking about, he will hit obstacles; when grasping for an object, he will miss it. Upon inquiry, he may explain that the light in the room is too dim or that he is not wearing his glasses. Also, the arousal reaction to opening of the eyes is missing in the EEG. Of course, visual evoked potentials (VEPs) show alteration of the late components. In many cases, there will be additional neurologic signs of brain stem dysfunction as well as alteration in brain stem evoked auditory responses (BEARs) and possibly also in the blink reflex because, in contrast to earlier teaching in neurology, there is not usually one single embolus occluding one single vessel, but rather a shower of emboli arriving in various branches of the basilar artery, in addition to occluding the top of it.

2.2 Toxic (Postangiographic)

Anton's syndrome is regularly found in *cortical blindness* resulting from transient toxic damage of the occipital lobes after angiography within the hindbrain circulation. This is a benign and not very frequent condition which usually clears within 1 or 2 days.

2.3 Psychogenic

Another important cause of acute blindness is an abnormal psychic reaction, formerly termed hysterical. The neurologic setting includes no features of the above-mentioned conditions: the patient reports that he can not see. Remarkably, he describes his surroundings as dark, whereas patients with organic cortical blindness are hard put to give a description of the absence of the visual experience. History is unremarkable in the neurologic sense, but will probably reveal a tendency to produce psychogenic symptoms in the past.

Pupillary reactions are normal. There are no brain stem signs. The patient will not be alarmed or desperate, but, like most hysterical patients, exhibit a certain "knowing" smile, which I have always found rather characteristic. Usually the EEG arousal reaction is present, and VEPs are normal.

The remaining diagnoses need no special discussion. One point however, is worth mentioning. Not infrequently, a patient has been amaurotic in one eye without being aware of it. If the good eye is affected by some prechiasmal disease, he may become blind, which confuses the diagnosis. In these instances, funduscopy and examination of the pupillary reactions to light are extremely helpful prior to the application of ancillary methods.

3 Acute Confusional State

In patients with acute confusional state the history is frequently rather fragmentary, if it is available at all. There are a particularly large number of diagnoses that have to be considered. Symptomatic therapy may obscure the picture and impede recognition of the underlying cause. Therefore, the various conditions should quickly be grouped in order to reduce the number of diagnostic options. Useful groupings are: toxic, inflammatory, vascular, metabolic, exacerbation of degenerative disease, traumatic, or postictal.

3.1 Alcoholic Withdrawal Syndrome

The most frequent intoxication is by alcohol. A confusional state due to excessive intake of alcohol is easily recognized. The full-blown picture of alcoholic withdrawal syndrome, i.e., the tremulous state, should not pose serious problems (see also Chap. 36). The case to be discussed here is the initial state of the withdrawal syndrome. These patients are usually anxious and agitated, disoriented as to time and place, and do not recognize their situation if they are invited to comment verbally on it. Strangely enough, however, they behave as other patients do and follow the doctor's and the nurse's instructions. Since the appearance of the withdrawal syndrome requires a long period of alcohol abuse, there will be tremor of the outstretched hands. The picture is completed by scleral jaundice and palpable liver. Among the laboratory findings, those indicating impairment of the hepatic synthesis processes are of greatest significance.

3.2 Drug Intoxication

Tranquilizing drugs may likewise produce intoxication, and thus disorientation. These patients, however, are not anxious or agitated, but rather present with diminished wakefulness. Ocular signs are helpful. Many drugs produce nystagmus and pupillary abnormalities (see Table 3.1). Tremor may be present, but not jaundice, and laboratory find-

Table 3.1. Ophthalmologic signs of intoxication

Ocular sign	Causative Factor
Miosis	Morphine derivatives
	Reserpine
	Meprobamate
	Acetylcholinesterase inhibitors
Mydriasis	Belladonna alkaloids
	Chlorperphenazine
	Imipramine
	Amitryptiline
	Botulism
	Cocain
Nystagmus	Barbiturates
	Benzodiazepines
	Phenytoin

ings are usually unremarkable. Drug intoxication is recognizable in the EEG, either by the appearance of frontal (barbiturates) or generalized (benzodiazepines) beta waves, or by dysrhythmic groupings mostly in the temporal leads. It is useful to send a urine specimen for toxicologic examination, but the procedure takes too much time to be of help on the spot. If the serum level of antiepileptic drugs can be assessed by enzymatic methods, this also applies to barbiturates and benzodiazepines, the most frequently used tranquilizing drugs. The same holds true for other psychotropic drugs, such as lithium. The results are available in half an hour at the most, and therapy can immediately be initiated.

3.3 Encephalitis

Another possibility which has to be taken into account if confusion has an acute onset is encephalitis. There need not be any illness prior to the outbreak of encephalitis. The leading signs, confusion and EEG alterations, are unfortunately quite unspecific. Neurologic findings may be unremarkable (for herpes simplex encephalitis, see Chaps. 14, 26, and 33). Fever need not be present, and CSF pleocytosis is not mandatory. If there is elevation of the protein level, this is quite a suggestive sign in the setting described here. Serological findings are available at the earliest after a week.

Frequently, the diagnosis has to be made by exclusion of other causes and observation, as well as a repeat examination, over the first few days. In the case of rapid deterioration of the patient, we therefore decide to start virostatic therapy even when serological confirmation is (still) missing.

3.4 Intracerebral Hemorrhage

The subgroup of vascular diseases includes various etiologies which are easily differentiated. While it is rare that ischemic stroke presents with predominantly psychiatric signs and symptoms (for an exception, see below), intracerebral hemorrhage may cause confusion prior to the appearance of hemiplegia or a brain stem syndrome. The diagnosis may be suspected if the patient has long-standing arterial hypertension. It cannot, however, be based on CSF findings. Gross focal plus general EEG alteration is suggestive, but definite proof can be obtained only by neuroimaging.

3.5 Subarachnoid Hemorrhage (SAH)

The onset of SAH is abrupt, and, as a rule, causes a headache the patient had never experienced prior to confusion. With very few exceptions, there is neck stiffness. Oculomotor and pupillomotor signs are frequent, and the lumbar tap produces blood-stained CSF that is xanthochromic after centrifugation.

3.6 Bilateral Posterior Artery Stroke

The patient is left blind, or nearly so, and frequently also confused by bilateral posterior artery stroke. In acute cortical blindness, anosognosia is almost the rule. These patients do not respond to purely visual stimuli; acoustic stimuli attract the gaze, but there is no precise fixation. Yet the patients deny being blind and describe their surroundings, when asked to do so, in a confabulatory way which adds to the confusion they may express spontaneously. Optokinetic nystagmus is absent. Details of the diagnostic procedure and the pertinent findings are given in Chap. 31.

9

3.7 Multi-Infarction Dementia

A series of minor (and sometimes major) strokes lead to chronic step-wise deterioration of various psychological functions, such as memory, word finding, and attention, to name but a few, in multi-infarction dementia. Frequently there are episodes of nocturnal confusion. Affectivity is flat, yet the patients are given to crying; sometimes there is pathologic laughter and crying.

At a given moment, another stroke leaves the patient in a state of confusion. The diagnosis is made on the basis of the characteristic history and of neurologic deficit attributable primarily to injury to the areas of supply of the middle cerebral artery. Neuroimaging shows the residua of previous strokes.

A variant of practical importance is encountered in the arteriosclerotic patients who do not have a history of multi-infarction dementia, but instead are well-balanced, reasonable elderly persons. Yet following a surgical intervention under general anesthesia, they wake up profoundly confused. This can also happen during an acute medical illness.

3.8 Alzheimer's Disease

In contrast, in Alzheimer's disease progression of neuropsychological deficit is steady. There are no sudden events. Neurologic signs are mild. Affective reactions are preserved, as is the social appearance of the patients. The onset of acute confusion is related to a change in the patient's life, such as moving, losing a dear member of the family, or admission to a hospital. Neuroimaging shows global reduction of cerebral volume.

3.9 Metabolic Derangement

An acute confusional state owing to metabolic derangement is almost impossible to diagnose on clinical grounds. It is true that flapping tremor, i.e., a tremor of increasing amplitude affecting predominantly proximal groups of muscles, is seen in hepatic and in renal failure. As a rule, however, the diagnosis is made on the basis of laboratory findings. It is therefore essential in the presence of an acute confusion of unknown etiology to ask for a large spectrum of laboratory examinations. A list of disease states, which is certainly not complete, includes: acute pancreatitis, Addison's disease, dehydration, hypercalcemia, hyperinsulinism, hyper- and hypoparathyroidism, porphyria, respiratory acidosis, sodium depletion, and thiamine deficiency.

3.10 Occult Bleeding (e.g., Intestinal Hemorrhage)

In this connection it should be mentioned that occult bleeding, e.g., intestinal hemorrhage, may reduce the quantity of circulating erythrocytes to such an extent that the result is global cerebral hypoxia, which manifests itself in confusion without neuropsychological signs or decrease in wakefulness.

3.11 Epileptic Twilight States

Twilight states resulting from epilepsy occur not only in patients who are known to have epilepsy, but also after the first seizure. They may follow a grand mal seizure or a series of these. In this case the patient is tense, disoriented, and does not correctly assess the situation. He may be paranoid, have a vague feeling of being threatened, and misinterpret even a neutral move of an other person. Consequently, he is likely to be aggressive in order to defend himself.

Aggressiveness does not result if the patient has an uninterrupted series of complex partial seizures. Frequently the patient acts slowly, performs inadequate actions, and gives the impression of not being fully awake. The diagnosis is greatly facilitated if there are oral automatisms like chewing, swallowing, smacking, and/or stereotypical movements of the hands, as frequently seen in a single partial complex seizure. The diagnosis is based on observation of the patient and EEG.

3.12 Post-traumatic Psychosis

The condition of post-traumatic psychosis is almost regularly misdiagnosed if the patient becomes psychotic after waking up from posttraumatic unconsciousness on the surgical ward. The characteristic features are anxiety, restlessness, and illusional misinterpretation of the surroundings, e.g., an infusion device is interpreted as a person threatening the patient. Patients are inclined to leave their bed or even the ward, in spite of strict admonitions to stay in bed. More often than not the condition is judged as misbehavior, and the pathologic nature of the state is not recognized.

4 Acute or Recurrent Headache

Headache is probably the most common complaint for which a patient consults any doctor. Inspection of the list, which is not even comprehensive, clearly shows that it would be pointless to submit this patient to examination by the technical machinery now available. He may request the doctor to do so, and may even be disappointed and mistrust the doctor instead of applauding him when he is informed, after a ten-minute inteview, that the symptoms which had prompted a year-long odyssey from one specialist to the next, including application of the most recent technological developments, are indicative of cluster headache, and are likely to respond favorably to lithium carbonate. The cost/efficiency relation is extremely unfavorable when the diagnostician relies on ancillary examinations in the search for the cause of headache. Instead, he should be aware of certain characteristic patterns in the patient's complaints, most of which can be verified within ten minutes.

4.1 Migraine

Most cases of migraine are diagnosed as "cranial neuritis," without a particular nerve being incriminated, or as trigeminal neuralgia (see below) and treated unsuccessfully with vitamins B_1 through B_{12}. The onset of symptoms usually occurs in early adulthood, but there are migrainous children, especially if there is a strong familial disposition. Some patients have their first bouts at or beyond the age of 40. The later the age of onset, the more important it is to look for a definite cause (so-called symptomatic migraine), such as an aneurysm or an arteriovenous angioma. This is not to say that every migrainous patient whose attacks start beyond the age of 40 should undergo cerebral angiography, but neuroimaging with contrast is as useful in these selected cases as it is superfluous in a migrainous teenager.

Family history is very revealing. Roughly 60% of migraine patients report, when questioned, similar attacks in other members of their family. Another important feature is the similarity of the recurrent attacks. At the beginning, the patient knows that the prodromal symptoms herald one of "his" attacks. Strangely enough, nevertheless rarely does he take a drug at this early stage when, in contrast to intake later on during the full-blown attack, it is likely to be of help.

These prodromata are frequently a certain uneasiness, a feeling of not waking up completely in the morning, or being unexplicably run down during the day in a way that is hard to describe. Some patients wake up at night with the headache they know so well, some have it when they wake up in the morning. Many claim they can tell what the weather is like without looking out of the window.

The typical signs and symptoms will not be described here in detail. Atypical features are frequent: unilateral headache (*hemi*crania) is by no means a sine qua non. Visual symptoms like "fortification scotomata" are of more theoretical than practical interest, and are rare. The important diagnostic clues are the following: positive family history; age of onset; recurrence, often in relation to some triggering event(s); duration (as a rule several hours or the entire day); and close similarity, if not identity, of symptoms. One should not expect each and every symptom described in the textbooks to occur in every patient; the important aspect is the general pattern. Complicated migraine is discussed in Chaps. 5 and 33, ophthalmoplegic migraine in Chap. 6.

4.2 Cluster Headache

It is appropriate to discuss cluster headache here, although in comparison to common migraine, the condition is less common and pathophysiology is still a matter of dispute. The typical attack starts at night with no recognizable triggering event, and some patients instinctively know what time it is when they awake with a strictly unilateral throbbing frontal headache. It frequently extends to the eyeball and rapidly increases in intensity to become almost intolerable. Rising and walking about helps a little. Usually, there is secretion from the lacrimal and nasal glands. Quite a few patients have miosis on the side of the headache, or even a full-blown Horner's syndrome. The attack is resistant to all common analgesics and lasts, as a rule, less than an hour. Unfortunately, it will recur several times during the night and the following day. It will awake the patient at the same hour the next night, and so on for a series of days or weeks: hence the term "cluster" headache. The condition is always "idiopathic," no ancillary examination will produce anything but false-positive signs, and treatment with injection of ergot derivatives or orally administered lithium carbonate usually helps within a few days.

4.3 Acute Glaucoma

Recurrent unilateral frontotemporal headache, mainly in the eye and beginning at night, is also characteristic of acute glaucoma. It does not end, though, after an hour. Also, the appearance of the patient should make confusion of the two states impossible: while in migraine, cluster headache, and, incidentally, also in trigeminal neuralgia (see below), the pupil shows unilateral miosis, in acute glaucoma there is fixed dilatation of the pupil, which leads to narrowing of the chamber angle and impedes the flow of aqueous humour. Conjunctival and ciliar congestion occurs in all three conditions, but is most pronounced in glaucoma. Of course, palpation of the globes shows a difference in intraocular pressure. Speedy diagnosis is essential, or the patient may lose his vision.

4.4 Trigeminal Neuralgia

Attacks of trigeminal neuralgia are so aptly described by the French term tic douloureux that they should not be confounded with any other condition. Of course, the patient will complain of constant pain in the upper or lower face, which does not always respect the area of supply of one or two of the branches of the trigeminal nerve as discretely as it should. On inquiry, however, he will admit that a longer (minutes, rarely hours) period of pain consists of series of very brief painful attacks ("tic") triggered by external stimuli such as eating, drinking, speaking, and touching the skin. These attacks make him suffer all the more, since he builds up a state of anxious expectation so that he can hardly avoid the triggering event(s). If he does so, he will have to refrain from speaking, eating, washing his face, brushing his teeth, and exposing himself to fresh air. The attacks can be stimulated by touching or pressing characteristic trigger zones roughly corresponding to the points of entrance of the three branches of the trigeminal nerve. Local anesthesia of these points helps temporarily, and at least abolishes the effect of stimulation of the trigger points. During the attacks, the vessels in the affected area are dilated. There is secretion from the lacrimal and nasal glands, and often there is miosis.

4.5 Cranial Arteritis

Unilateral frontal headache is reported by patients of about 60 years of age or more, who suffer from cranial arteritis, which was formerly called frontal or temporal arteritis. This is a giant-cell arteritis of autoimmune origin, affecting widespread territories in the distribution of the external and internal carotid arteries – hence the new, more appropriate term. Patients report a persistent, throbbing, temporal headache. Since not only the superficial temporal artery is affected, they also report a unique symptom which is termed "intermittent claudication of mastication." This is pain in the masseter muscles which develops on chewing. The mechanism is the same as that involved in intermittent claudication of gait: a process of arterial stenosis prevents the increase in blood supply needed for muscular activity.

While the much-reported thickening and pulselessness of the superficial temporal artery develops only in an advanced stage of the disease – usually in the 2nd week – characteristic laboratory findings can be obtained right at the onset of the symptoms: extreme acceleration of erythrocyte sedimentation rate, anemia, leukocytosis, increase in α_2-globulin, and serum IgG. Early diagnosis is mandatory, because early treatment with corticosteroids followed by long-term application of azathioprine can virtually stop the course of the disease, whereas belated diagnosis carries the risk of unilateral blindness and hemiplegia. The diagnosis is confirmed by biopsy of the superficial temporal artery, which reveals giant-cell arteritis.

For association with *polymyalgia rheumatica*, see Chap. 23.

4.6 Subarachnoid Hemorrhage (SAH)

The development of symptoms and signs in SAH (see also Chaps. 19 and 31) is quite characteristic, so it is very puzzling that in most instances the diagnosis is missed and valuable time is lost. Virtually all patients report sudden or rapid onset of headache, not necessarily in the occipital region, which they have never experienced before. The sudden onset of a headache of unprecedented severity is the leading and frequently the only complaint; all other symptoms and signs may be absent, and consciousness may be preserved. Oculomotor signs, e.g., third nerve paralysis, give valuable clues to localization (posterior communicating artery), but should not be expected in all or even the majority of cases. Even neck stiffness may be absent, although the patient is wholly conscious. Epileptic fits occur in rare instances and are mainly due to intracerebral hemorrhage.

Lumbar puncture will show sanguinolent CSF, which upon centrifugation is xanthochromic 6 h or more after the event. Neuroimaging will show the extent, sometimes even the source, of the bleeding. This is clearly a case for emergency admission to the nearest department of neurology or neurosurgery, where diagnosis is verified by cerebral angiography. Medical and surgical treatment will not be described here in detail.

The spectrum of erroneous diagnoses and consecutive inappropriate treatment procedures is most distressing. Meningitis or acute deterioration of a posterior fossa brain tumor are "reasonable" errors, because these would lead to early hospital admission. No excuse can be given for attributing the alarming cranial symptoms to cervical spondylosis, and the consequent application of chiropractic manipulations which might provoke recurrent bleeding with fatal outcome. Also, injection of local anesthetics into the C-2 segments under the assumption of "occipital neuralgia" has no defensible basis. Every doctor should be aware that cervical spondylosis affects the levels C-5 through C-8 with increasing frequency, and that the ensuing pain will not radiate to the neck or head, but rather to the shoulder and arm(s). If there is vertebral disease affecting the uppermost segments of the column with occipital radiation of pain, it is certainly not degenerative, but rather malignant or inflammatory in nature, and requires thorough radiological and medical diagnostic measures before any therapeutic procedures other than the application of analgesics are introduced.

4.7 Painful Diabetic Ophthalmoplegia

It is easy to mistake painful ophthalmoplegia for SAH. In elderly diabetic patients it occurs as acute partial or complete paralysis of the somatic fibers of the third nerve, accompanied by pain in the upper half of the face. In contrast to SAH, the visceral fibers are not affected, which provides an important diagnostic clue. Also, there is no neck stiffness and wakefulness is preserved.

Most patients have a history of diabetes mellitus. Muscular reflexes are frequently diminished or absent, at least in the leg, and vibration is felt as continuous pressure on the ankles and toes. No additional examinations are necessary in these cases. Prognosis is fair, with recovery to be expected over a period of 1–3 months. Painful diabetic ophthalmoplegia is one of the manifestations of diabetic neuropathy. Since the third nerve does not contain sensory fibers, one has to assume additional damage to the ophthalmic, and sometimes also to the maxillary, branch of the trigeminal nerve. Absence of pupillary dilatation or of paralysis of accommodation is somewhat surprising, because other variants of diabetic neuropathy quite regularly include affection of visceral fibers (see also Chap. 34).

4.8 Tolosa-Hunt Syndrome

Another instance of painful ophthalmoplegia is seen in Tolosa-Hunt syndrome. Again, it is mainly patients of middle or advanced age who are affected. Over a period of several days, partial or total unilateral ophthalmoplegia develops, and the patient experiences severe pain in the area of supply of the ophthalmic nerve. Frequently, there are signs of vascular congestion in the affected eye, and there may be protrusion of the bulb. The combination of signs and symptoms strongly points to a disease process localized at the tip of the orbit or in the cavernous sinus. The diagnosis of Tolosa-Hunt syndrome, which is a granulomatous retro-orbital inflammatory process, is made more often than not by excluding all other differential diagnoses. Corticosteroids, as a rule, lead to a rapid amelioration of signs and symptoms, but relapses are frequent if the treatment is discontinued.

4.9 Herpes Zoster Ophthalmicus

The onset of herpes zoster ophthalmicus may consist solely of frontal headache, which lasts for several days before the appearance of the typical eruption.

4.10 Post-Lumbar-Puncture Headache

Headache frequently occurs after a lumbar puncture. Typically, it increases when the patient assumes the erect, and decreases when he resumes the supine, position. Many patients complain of an unspecified droning noise, which they localize within the head. Some complain of nausea, some develop a minor degree of neck stiffness. Prognosis is good. It helps if the doctor can convince the patient that a resolution may be expected within a few days.

If the condition appears spontaneously, one might feel obliged to perform a lumbar tap under the suspected diagnosis of lymphocytic meningitis. One will find low CSF pressure, sometimes to the extent that no CSF can be obtained. If the Queckenstedt maneuver yields some fluid, it usually has a normal cell count and a slightly elevated protein level. Unfortunately, the diagnostic lumbar puncture will increase the patient's symptoms, which are felt to be caused by a temporarily diminished production of CSF and not by loss of total CSF volume within the CNS (normal daily production is 500 ml).

4.11 Arterial Hypertension and Incipient Stroke

Recurrent headache is a frequent sign of arterial hypertension, especially in the initial stage of the disease. In these cases, it is mandatory to measure blood pressure several times a day, under various conditions. Also, incipient stroke may begin with unilateral headache. It is useful to know that headache occurring prior to hemiplegia is not necessarily a symptom suggesting brain tumor.

4.12 Psychogenic, Depressive

So far the discussion was centered on disease states which physically threaten the patient's health. The majority of patients seeking medical advice for headache, however, have psychogenic pain. The range of symptoms extends from chronic or relapsing depressive illness to reaction to a conflict where the patient sees no alternative to outright simulation, sometimes a variant of Münchhausen's syndrome. In the German literature a most disagreeable variant is described, the Koryphaenkiller syndrome, which might be described as a condition in which a person of hysterical personality structure in the serious sense of the term endeavours to confuse the diagnostician in a conscious or unconscious kind of "one-upmanship." The symptoms and signs he presents do not fit a known pattern, so the doctor sooner or later has to admit defeat, to the great satisfaction of the patient. In the case of Koryphaenkiller syndrome it is advisable not to be defensive or to feel humiliated, but rather to calmly admit that unfortunately medicine has to the best of our knowledge no cure for these symptoms.

Whatever variant of psychic pain be present, it is of the utmost importance not to lose sight of the common experience that pain, and in particular headache, frequently has no somatic cause. More often than not the situation will be clarified if the doctor encourages the patient to report on his personal life and anxieties.

5 Acute Hemiplegia

5.1 Stroke

Faced with a patient who has suffered acute hemiplegia, the doctor will usually assume that this is an instance of stroke. Stroke occurs, of course, not only in the elderly arteriopathic patient, but also in juvenile or young adult persons. In these latter cases one should consider cardiogenic embolism or one of the rare vascular diseases like fibromuscular dysplasia, or rheumatic or syphilitic angiitis.

Prior to these considerations, one should try to find out whether this is a case of ischemic or hemorrhagic stroke, or whether there is venous thrombosis. This latter condition is discussed in Chap. 14.

Unfortunately, there is no way of distinguishing between ischemic and hemorrhagic stroke other than neuroimaging. All other indirect evidence referred to in the textbooks is most unreliable. Furthermore, the seemingly unitary subgroup of ischemic stroke is caused either by hemidynamic failure due to extracranial arterial stenosis, or by cardiac embolism, or by arterio-arterial embolism originating in an ulcerative extra- or intracerebral plaque, or by local thrombosis of a small arterial vessel. These different kinds of stroke require differential treatment.

5.2 Complicated Migraine

In juvenile and young adult patients complicated migraine is an important alternative. This is a variant of migraine in which transient focal signs like hemiplegia, aphasia, or hemianopia occur prior to the unilateral headache, which, like other characteristic symptoms of migraine, may be only minor.

The diagnosis is relatively easy when there is a family and/or personal history of recurrent headache. If the history is unremarkable, there is a pathognomonic combination of signs and symptoms consisting of severe neurologic deficit and very pronounced focal EEG abnormality in the presence of normal neuroimaging results.

One may rely on this triad, however, only when it is certain that signs and symptoms are due to hemispheric dysfunction. If the migraine occurs in the territory of the hindbrain (i.e., vertebrobasilar) circulation, normal neuroimaging results are of no diagnostic help, and EEG abnormality may be absent, or minor and bilateral. Here, Doppler ultrasound study of the vertebral arteries is of great value, because high-grade stenosis or occlusion in the vertebrobasilar system is extremely rare in the presence of normal ultrasound findings. In case of doubt, angiography should definitely be undertaken, rather than risk failure to diagnose a treatable vascular lesion (see Chap. 31).

5.3 Brain Tumor

The first sign of brain tumor may be acute hemiplegia, and the reason, as a rule, is bleeding into the tumor or the surrounding tissue from rapidly formed nutrient vessels with deficient arterial walls. Progression of neurologic deficit and decreasing vigilance, together with signs of general hemispheric dysfunction, such as grasping and groping reflexes, are quite characteristic of "apoplectic glioma."

5.4 Encephalitis

It is not well-known that in roughly 10% of cases the onset of encephalitis resembles a stroke. Usually, the relentless deterioration, with clouding of consciousness, grasping and groping reflexes, and additional symptoms that cannot be localized in the territory of a major artery or a branch thereof will provoke ancillary examinations. The EEG shows widespread abnormality, neuroimaging is normal during the first few days, and CSF shows mild pleocytosis and an only slightly elevated protein level, with normal or elevated lactate level.

5.5 Postictal State

As mentioned in Chap. 14, an *epileptic seizure* may go unnoticed, and in the case of focal origin the patient will be comatose or confused, with hemiplegia. The usual signs found after a grand mal seizure are described in Chap. 31. The EEG frequently shows "epileptic" activity also after a seizure. Partial seizures with Todd's paralysis are reported by the patient if he is not aphasic. The search for the underlying cause of epilepsy with hemiplegia follows the guidelines given in Chap. 16.

5.6 Diabetic Metabolic Derangement

Acute hemiplegia may be caused by diabetes mellitus under two conditions. In *nonketotic hyperosmolar* metabolic derangement hemiplegia is frequent. The EEG shows focal plus general abnormality, but neuro-imaging and ultrasound studies are normal. Diagnosis is made on the basis of laboratory tests, which should be applied freely in acute hemiplegia of unknown etiology. With adequate therapy, signs and symptoms resolve rapidly. Hypoglycemia leads not only to convulsions and confusion, but also to hemiplegia. The diagnostic clues described in the preceding paragraphs also apply here.

5.7 Multiple Sclerosis

The presence of multiple sclerosis should be suspected in young individuals especially when there is sensorimotor hemiplegia with ataxia, and when vigilance is well preserved. The EEG frequently shows little alteration, and neuroimaging reveals an area of hypodensity which does not correspond to a vascular territory, nor is it, as a rule, a space-occupying lesion. Evoked potentials may not be indicative of multiple CNS lesions. CSF findings are diagnostic if IgG production within the CNS is demonstrated, but unfortunately, CSF may be normal during the first bout(s), or nearly so. In these cases, the correct diagnosis will be provided only by a follow-up study.

6 Acute Paralysis of Extraocular Muscle(s)

The table indicates that acute diplopia cannot be dismissed as a trivial event. It is true that in large statistical surveys a strikingly high proportion of patients are classified as having diplopia of unknown etiology, and that the paralysis resolves with or without therapy over a period of roughly 3 months. The recognizable causes, however, are conditions for which there is a specific and successful treatment.

6.1 Myasthenia Gravis

Proptosis and/or diplopia may be the first sign of myasthenia gravis. In this case, the characteristic fatigue upon exercise is not yet present in the limb muscles, or at least the patient is not aware of it. History may or may not reveal that the signs and symptoms become more severe during the day and are less severe in the morning. Often one can demonstrate weakness on exercise by asking the patient to open and close his eyes forcefully 30 times, or by requiring him to follow repeatedly the examiner's fingers in the main directions of conjugate gaze (lateral, vertical, and transverse). To this end, one can also elicit optokinetic nystagmus for half a minute, which is easily done by means of a portable drum bearing alternating black and white stripes or a ruler. If there is an increase in signs and symptoms, their reversibility should be demonstrated by intravenous injection of a substance that blocks the activity of cholinesterase, i.e., the enzyme that breaks down the neuromuscular transmitter, acetylcholine. Since these substances (edrophonium hydrochloride; physostigmine) increase not only the somatic but also the autonomic effects of acetylcholine, 0.5 mg of atropine should be given intravenously prior to the test dose.

Whatever the result of these tests, it is advisable to apply stimulation EMG to limb muscles with a view to demonstrating the characteristic decrement in the amplitude of action potentials, which can also be reversed by the pharmacologic tests described above.

Stimulation EMG has two purposes: first, it is important to know whether the patient has purely ocular myasthenia or generalization to limb muscles. In the latter case the patient is a candidate for thymectomy, provided he meets the medical and surgical criteria for operative treatment. Second, Eaton-Lambert syndrome, a paraneoplastic condition imitating myasthenia gravis, can be recognized by a typical EMG pattern: the amplitude of action potentials shows waxing and waning during stimulation, in contrast to waning alone in myasthenia (see also Chap. 40).

6.2 Congenital Aneurysms of the Circle of Willis

Congenital aneurysms are mainly located on the anterior part of the circle of Willis; hence, the most frequent neurologic indication as to localization is unilateral paralysis of the extraocular muscles. The third cranial nerve is usually affected. The most common cause is SAH, diagnosis of which is discussed in Chap. 4. In very rare instances diplopia and/or proptosis is caused by temporary swelling of the aneurysm, and this condition is termed paralytic aneurysm. Diagnosis is very difficult, because there are so many other causes of extraocular paralysis that few clinicians will subject these patients to cerebral angiography. Sometimes the aneurysm is visualized by neuroimaging, especially when it is large and partially thrombosed.

6.3 Spontaneous or Traumatic Carotis-Cavernosus Fistula

Since all nerves supplying the extraocular muscles run through the cavernous sinus, any disease state with this location is likely to produce acute diplopia. Of greatest significance is a fistula between the internal carotid artery and the cavernous sinus. These fistulas arise following head trauma, and sometimes become symptomatic with a latency of many weeks. They also occur spontaneously, probably by rupture of a small arteriosclerotic aneurysm. In most instances the first (ophthalmic) branch of the trigeminal nerve is also affected, and the patient has local pain in the front and/or eye, which does not have the characteristics of trigeminal neuralgia (see Chap. 4).

The diagnosis is greatly facilitated when the patient complains of a rhythmic bruit that is synchronous with his heart beat and diminishes in volume when the ipsilateral carotid artery is compressed. On close inspection pulsating veins in the medial angle of the eye can sometimes be recognized. With the help of a periorbital Doppler study it is possible to demonstrate the greatly increased flow in the supratrochlear and angular veins, and subsequent angiography confirms the diagnosis.

6.4 Parasellar Disease (Tumor, Granuloma)

Other disease states of parasellar localization, such as tumor or granuloma, can be recognized only by neuroimaging plus angiography.

6.5 Diabetic Ophthalmoplegia

An important alternative to the paralytic aneurysm is diabetic ophthalmoplegia. In most instances onset is acute, and there is incomplete third nerve palsy accompanied by ipsilateral pain in the forehead. The patients never develop neck stiffness. Also, the paralysis spares the autonomic fibers, and thus the pupil is not dilated, in contrast to third nerve palsy caused by aneurysm, where, as a rule, the autonomic fibers are affected. As in all diabetic neuropathies, the patient is not necessarily frankly diabetic. Quite frequently, one can demonstrate only reduced tolerance to orally administered glucose solution.

6.6 Ocular Myositis

There are two variants of ocular myositis. In the first, acute exophthalmic myositis, there are, in addition to paralysis of multiple extraocular muscles, all the possible signs of inflammatory disease of the eye. These include hyperemia of the conjunctival and ciliar vessels, pain which increases on any attempt to move the eye ball, and the acute inflammatory condition as indicated by laboratory tests. Chronic myositis is not so easily recognized. Neuroimaging is a most powerful tool, in that it demonstrates increased thickness of the extraocular muscles. This is also the case in *thyrotoxic ophthalmopathy*. *Tumor* and (inflammatory) *pseudotumor* of the orbital cavity are also recognized by neuroimaging.

6.7 Tolosa-Hunt Syndrome

A rare condition is Tolosa-Hunt Syndrome, a granulomatous process at the tip of the orbit. Diagnosis requires orbitophlebography and carotid angiography (see also Chap. 4).

6.8 Cranial Arteritis

The symptoms cranial arteritis are temporal pain; thickening of the temporal artery, which eventually becomes pulseless; ischemic pain in the masseter muscles upon chewing; and the "inflammatory constellation" revealed by laboratory tests (see also Chap. 4).

6.9 Ischemic Brain Stem Lesions

Dysfunction of the nuclei of either the third, fourth, or sixth nerve, or a combination of these, is caused by brain stem lesions of various etiologies. The most common cause is circumscribed ischemia in the territory of the penetrating paramedian branches of the basilar artery. The diagnosis is suggested when there is acute onset of signs and symptoms in an elderly patient who has other signs of generalized atherosclerosis. A history of instances of brain stem dysfunction gives an important clue. More often than not, ultrasound examination is unremarkable, as is angiography of the hindbrain circulation, because the small brain stem vessels are not visualized. Brain stem hemorrhage is diagnosed by neuroimaging.

6.10 Metastatic Brain Stem Lesions

The most frequent location of metastatic brain stem lesions is the midbrain level, where they lead to third nerve palsy or paralysis of upward gaze. They may be visualized by neuroimaging with contrast or by angiography. More frequently, the diagnosis is made by follow-up examination, which reveals progression of the symptoms and, in particular, bilateral affection of the cranial nerves.

6.11 Multiple Sclerosis

Brain stem lesions lead to acute diplopia also in multiple sclerosis. The diagnosis is easy if previous bouts have affected other parts of the CNS, and thus the requirements of multiplicity in time and space are met (see also Chap. 10). If diplopia heralds the disease, not only history but also results of ancillary examinations (evoked potentials, neuroimaging, lumbar tap) may be unremarkable. It is wise to be reticent if one suspects multiple sclerosis to be the cause of transient diplopia, because nothing is gained by raising an alarm that may turn out to be false or at least premature.

6.12 Wernicke's Encephalopathy

Vitamin B_1 deficiency causes Wernicke's encephalopathy in heavy drinkers who either have an intestinal malabsorption syndrome or have given up regular intake of food. Other causes are of no practical significance, with one important exception: there are patients in intensive care units who are fed intravenously for periods of weeks with large amounts of carbohydrates. Wernicke's encephalopathy ensues when the vitamin supply is insufficient and the increased metabolism of carbohydrates leads to vitamin B_1 depletion.

The classic triad consists of third nerve palsy [somatic and autonomic, i.e., with dilated pupil(s)], nystagmus and cerebellar ataxia, and decreased vigilance. The latter is not required for diagnosis but ocular symptoms are invariably present, and cerebellar ataxia is frequent. Onset may be quite acute, and the dramatic amelioration following parenteral supply of vitamin B_1 (100 mg daily) is diagnostic.

6.13 Meningitis (Carcinomatous, Tuberculous, Sarcoidosis, Fungous, Other)

Peripheral lesion of one or more of the nerves supplying the extraocular muscles can, of course, also indicate a disease process affecting the *leptomeninges*. The patients do not necessarily present with a meningitic syndrome. Tuberculous meningitis, sarcoidosis, fungous meningitis, or carcinomatosis may all take a mild course that merely gives the patient a general appearance of being ill until diplopia points to participation of the nervous system in the disease. In these cases a lumbar tap will decide the diagnosis, provided all available CSF examinations have been requested by the doctor. Sometimes repeat examination is necessary.

6.14 Pregnancy

Finally, there are instances of lesions of cranial nerves in pregnancy, the pathogenesis of which is not fully understood, but the outcome of which is usually favorable. This diagnosis, however, can be made only by exclusion, because pregnancy gives no protection against any of the disease states discussed above.

6.15 Ophthalmoplegic Migraine

Recurrent ophthalmoplegia with headache lasting 1 or 2 h is sometimes diagnosed as ophthalmoplegic migraine. The existence of this variant of migraine, however, is considered doubtful by many authorities, and it might well be that most, if not all, cases belong to one of the categories discussed above.

7 Acute Unilateral Seventh Nerve (Facial) Palsy

It is a traditional error in neurology to distinguish between central and peripheral seventh nerve palsy. Textbooks go to great pains to explain that the frontal muscles receive bilateral innervation, and that frowning is therefore still possible in "central facial paralysis." There is some uncertainty about closure of the eye, and it is generally assumed that while the eyelids are wider in "central paralysis," closure of the eye is preserved.

All this is true as far as clinical observation is concerned, but it does not make physiological sense. The reader will remember Hughlings Jackson's famous dictum that the brain (i.e., the cortex) does not know of nerves, it knows only of movements. One would not call a wristdrop resulting from stroke a central paralysis of the radial nerve, or a foot-drop of subcortical origin a central peroneal paralysis. Closer observation clearly shows that in all three instances there is more involved than just weakness of muscles supplied by one peripheral nerve when disease affects central motor pathways.

7.1 Idiopathic (Cryptogenic)

The most common cause of acute unilateral seventh nerve palsy is called idiopathic or Bell's palsy. It must be more than coincidental that in a great proportion of cases the patient has been exposed to a draft of some sort, yet the exact role of a "refrigeratory" insult to the nerve remains to be established. Viral etiology has many advocates.

If the weakness becomes complete during the first 2 days or so, a fast and satisfactory recovery is rather unlikely. In an incomplete paralysis one may safely predict a good outcome. Pain has no prognostic significance, and affection of the gustatory or lacrimal fibers and of the small branch to the tensor tympani muscle, giving rise to hyperacusis, does not indicate the level of damage in the fallopian canal, but in the diameter of the nerve.

7.2 Ear Conditions

It is advisable to examine the mastoid bone and the tympanic membrane, because all kinds of ear conditions, including mastoiditis, may damage the facial nerve, and these are frequently recognized by signs of inflammation or by a perforated tympanic membrane. Along the same lines, x-rays of the petrous bone and of the squama temporalis may reveal local destructive or inflammatory disease. Lack of pneumatization is frequently associated with recurrent inflammatory disease of the middle ear.

7.3 Tumor of the Cerebellopontine Angle

Also, x-ray may show enlargement of the internal auditory meatus owing to a tumor in the cerebellopontine angle. These tumors are, of course, better visualized by neuroimaging, but given their relatively low frequency and the even lower frequency of facial palsy as their first sign, it would be exaggerated to require neuroimaging in every case of acute unilateral seventh nerve palsy.

7.4 Herpes Zoster Oticus

The comment that pain has no prognostic significance requires one qualification. In herpes zoster oticus, the facial palsy may be accompanied or preceded by pain in the meatus acusticus externus or in the area of the tympanic membrane. Again, inspection of these regions is very helpful, because the typical herpetic efflorescences are sometimes hidden deep in the external ear. Other nerves that are affected in herpes zoster are the fifth, the eighth (vertigo, tinnitus), and, in rare instances, virtually every cranial nerve down to the twelfth. Prognosis is poor for recovery from the facial palsy.

7.5 Traumatic Facial Palsy

Facial palsy of traumatic origin is mostly seen when there is a fracture of the petrous bone. In longitudinal fracture there is no need for surgical therapy, because prognosis is usually good. In transverse fracture, which is often accompanied (or recognized) by hematotympanum, prognosis is poor, and surgical therapy is indicated.

7.6 Meningitis

The seventh nerve, and many other cranial nerves, may be affected by meningitis of various etiologies. One should bear in mind that the onset of meningitis with paralysis of the cranial nerves is quite characteristic of *tuberculous meningitis* and of *sarcoidosis*. Mild lymphocytic or granulocytic pleocytosis, relatively high protein and low glucose, in contrast to high lactate, levels constitute a very suggestive constellation. Since direct demonstration of *Mycobacterium tuberculosis* is an exception, the decision to begin tuberculostatic therapy must be taken as soon as the disease is suspected.

7.7 Polyneuritis

It is well known that facial palsy may occur during ascending polyneuritis of the *Guillain-Barré* type. In these instances it is essential to observe the patient for signs of respiratory distress, that is, to be prepared to provide artificial respiration and to examine the patient repeatedly for preservation of the reactivity of cardiac frequency to alteration in respiratory frequency or pressure on the ocular bulbs. This is because a lack of reactivity indicates that the patient requires an external demand pacemaker. More important is the consideration that in rare cases polyneuropathy may be of the descending variant, i.e., starting with facial palsy and affecting limb (and respiratory and/or autonomic) nerves during the first week. Here, it is advisable to examine the patient regularly for the level of proprioceptive reflexes.

7.8 Diabetes and Pregnancy

Two rarer factors that predispose to facial palsy are diabetes and pregnancy, and these conditions are easily recognized if looked for.

7.9 Melkersson-Rosenthal Syndrome

Recurrent unilateral facial palsy does occur even in the "idiopathic" variant. It is, however, more suggestive of Melkersson-Rosenthal syndrome. In this rare condition facial palsy is accompanied by swelling of the lips and tongue owing to local granulomatous inflammation. Etiology is unknown, but steroid therapy is of some help.

7.10 Pontine Lesions

Finally, seventh nerve palsy may also have its origin in a lesion of the facial nucleus. Pontine lesions, as a rule, are not limited to one nucleus, but affect neighboring fiber tracts and nuclei. Apart from careful neurologic examination, localization and extent of these brain stem lesions can be assessed by electrophysiological studies, such as the blink reflex. Excitation of the reflex arch travels on the afferent side via fifth nerve fibers and utilizes a rather complex system of wiring within the brain stem, while the efferent pathway is via the seventh nerve. Other methods are brain stem auditory evoked responses (BAER) and somatosensory evoked potentials (SSEPs).

8 Brown-Séquard's Syndrome

(Mostly Cervical Localization)

The Brown-Séquard syndrome is one of neurology's classics, which, however, is more notorious in textbooks than in medical reality. It is indicative of circumscribed damage to one half of the spinal cord, and occurs mostly at the lower cervical or midthoracic level. On the side of the lesion there is central paresis of the ipsilateral limb or limbs (depending on the level of damage) and impairment of touch and "deep sensation," e.g., temporal discrimination of successive local stimuli or awareness of joint movements. Contralaterally there is loss or impairment of sensation of pain and temperature.

8.1 Multiple Sclerosis

The most common cause is multiple sclerosis, at least if the patient is below the age of 60. In this instance, as a rule, the syndrome evolves acutely. Rarely will this particular spinal manifestation be the first event of the illness. The history is likely to reveal periods of numbness in distal parts of the limbs, bladder problems, impairment of gait, and diplopia or blurred vision, to name but a few characteristic signs of the disease. Incidentally, multiple sclerosis is one of the diagnoses that can be made with great certainty by careful history taking alone. Many patients suspect they may have the disease and will sooner or later begin to question the doctor. He should not hesitate, but should rather help the patient to face reality and explain that the prognosis is better than believed by most patients and their relatives.

Neurologic examination may reveal sequelae of previous bouts, such as missing abdominal reflexes or pallor of the optic discs. Today, the most conclusive diagnostic measure is the electrophysiological examination. Alterations in the amplitude, form, and latency of the visual evoked potentials (VEPs) contribute the most (about 90%), followed by the somatosensory evoked potentials (SSEPs). This is not surprising, given the length of the pathways transmitting the signals through the spinal cord and brain stem. A similar consideration holds true for the blink reflex, the afferent signals of which are transmitted via the trigeminal, and the efferent via the facial, nerve with a widespread area of interconnection within the lower brain stem.

It is not always necessary to examine the CSF, but if this is done the evidence of local IgG production within the CNS is virtually diagnostic. If the patient refuses lumbar puncture I do not, as a rule, insist, because the diagnostic gain is limited, and early diagnosis has more social consequences than medical benefits. Neuroimaging may show an overall loss of brain volume or areas of demyelination not identical with areas of vascular supply.

8.2 Syndrome of the Anterior Spinal Artery
(Primary Vascular Disease or Secondary to Spinal Tumor)

In the elderly, vascular disease of the spinal cord may occasionally lead to Brown-Séquard's syndrome instead of the full-blown syndrome of the anterior spinal artery. In this case, there is ischemia in one of the small penetrating sulcocommissural branches of the anterior spinal artery, which enter the cord alternatingly in the left or right half of a given segment, usually at the midthoracic level. Onset is acute. The syndrome may be only partial, so that the patient is still ambulatory when seen by the doctor. A purely vascular origin of the spinal insult is rightly suspected when this is a typical "vascular" patient with a history of coronary insufficiency, bruits over the arteries in the inguinal area, and weak or missing pulses of the dorsal pedal arteries.

Yet even in this seemingly unequivocal case, it is important to establish whether the vascular syndrome is caused by arterio-arterial embolism, high-grade stenosis of one of the arteries feeding the spinal cord, or a space-occupying lesion compromising the circulation in the anterior spinal or sulco-commissural arteries. In the latter case the patient may have complained for a certain period of time of girdle pain which may be worsened by coughing and is regrettably often treated as a symptom of spinal spondylosis, which for biomechanical reasons is extremely rare and usually asymptomatic at the thoracic level. The patient may have developed a stiff and slow way of walking, which is often erroneously diagnosed and treated as parkinsonism. Bladder problems are likely to be considered as being of prostatic origin. Also, local back pain is not usually a symptom of spinal vascular disease.

The sequence of diagnostic measures applied in my department is as follows: after history taking and neurologic examination, which may provide important clues to diagnosis, plain x-ray examination of the relevant part of the vertebral column and emergency blood tests are performed at the same time. If there is destruction of a vertebra and the patient does not yet have a complete transverse syndrome of the spinal cord, we proceed to myelography. Myelography, of course, is also done if plain x-ray is normal and yet there is suspicion of a space-occupying spinal lesion. In our experience, spinal CT and myelography are not alternatives, but rather two examinations that complement each other very favorably. CT myelography, that is, spinal CT after intrathecal application of contrast material, is most revealing at the cervical and thoracic levels. It provides not only a precise localization of the lesion, but also CSF findings, and, finally, permits visualization of the region(s) adjacent to the vertebral column.

No time should be lost should surgical intervention prove necessary, as the neurosurgeon must operate on the patient before a complete transverse syndrome of the spinal cord develops.

8.3 Lateral Disc Herniation

I have seen several cases of cervical Brown-Séquard's syndrome due to a herniated cervical disc. One occurred while the patient was stretching out his arms in the morning, lying in bed in hospital waiting to be examined for the cause of radicular brachial pain. This kind of pain and/or paresthesia, a field where the problems are all too frequently underestimated, will be dealt with separately in Chap. 25. Suffice it to say here that an event such as that described above should prompt immediate x-ray examination of the vertebral column, followed by cervical myelography via the lateral approach to C-1 to C-2. This resolves the situation in less than half an hour. One final word of caution: not every herniated disc is preceded by a history of typical complaints.

The diagnostic steps in the case of vertebral tumor or extradural lymphoma or the like are not discussed here in detail because they are beyond the scope of this book.

9 Burning Feet and Restless Legs

These two conditions are described under the same general heading because both are, in most instances, indicative of polyneuropathy. The term "burning feet" is self-explanatory. The burning pain is felt permanently, although it increases during the night, when there is less distracting external stimulation. Some patients describe pain as being localized specifically on the plantar aspect of the foot, some experience burning throughout the foot. "Restless legs" is a term the Swedish author Ekbom tried to explain by the Latin wording *anxietas tibiarum*. During the day the patients are relatively well, but as soon as they are in bed, and with increasing intensity during the night, they feel an irresistible urge to move the legs under the cover, sometimes to the extent that they have to get up.

Motor symptoms are scarce. Frequently, there is no weakness or atrophy, and reflexes may be normal. There need not be sensory loss for any given kind of stimulus.

9.1 Burning Feet Syndrome

Polyneuropathy of toxic, nutritional, or metabolic origin involves burning feet syndrome.

9.1.1 Toxic Polyneuropathy

The most common toxic polyneuropathies are due to ingestion or inhalation of heavy metal compounds. This occurs either in certain professions (occupational diseases) or in suicide attempts. Homicidal application of heavy metals has become quite rare. Common agents are lead, thallium (insecticides), arsenic, and mercury. Also, various drugs may cause polyneuropathy with burning feet syndrome.

The important point is not to dismiss the patient's complaint as psychogenic, but to recognize the syndrome as characteristic of organic damage to the peripheral nervous system. This recognition should prompt the doctor to inquire about personal and social history, and to apply electrophysiological (EMG and nerve conduction) studies. Neurologic findings are frequently normal. The characteristic electrophysiological finding is that of axonal damage, i.e., muscular denervation in the presence of relatively normal nerve conduction.

9.1.2 Nutritional Deficiency Polyneuropathy
Another less frequent cause is nutritional deficiency polyneuropathy. The syndrome has been described in deficiency of vitamins B_1, B_2, B_6, and B_{12} in the malabsorption syndrome and in alcohol abuse. It has not yet been determined whether damage to the peripheral nervous system in alcoholic patients depends entirely on nutritional deficiency or whether the toxic action of alcohol is also operative.

9.1.3 Polyneuropathy in Metabolic Disorder
Among the metabolic causes, diabetes is of the greatest importance. Amyloidosis and macroglobulinemia are rarer conditions.

9.2 Restless Legs Syndrome

In many instances, restless legs syndrome is indicative of polyneuropathy. However, roughly half of the cases are unexplained and should potentially be considered psychogenic after careful and repeat examination.

9.2.1 Chronic Anemia
Restless legs may be caused by chronic anemia, and there need not be gross signs of polyneuropathy, either on neurologic or electrophysiological examination.

9.2.2 Chronic Renal Failure
Restless legs syndrome may be caused by chronic renal failure prior to the recognition of polyneuropathy. This condition, again, is first detected in nerve conduction studies, long before there is weakness, alteration of reflexes, or "objective" sensory loss.

9.2.3 Diabetic and Other Metabolic Diseases of the Peripheral Nerves
The syndrome may also be caused by diabetic and other metabolic diseases of the peripheral nerves. Most of these diseases lead to impairment in nerve conduction and are thus detected by conduction velocity studies long before there is any clinical indication of polyneuropathy.

9.2.4 Alcoholic Neuropathy

Restless legs are also reported in alcoholic neuropathy, but this connection is certainly rare.

9.2.5 Paraneoplastic Polyneuropathy

More common is the connection of paraneoplastic polyneuropathy with the restless legs syndrome. As in all paraneoplastic affections of the nervous system, the underlying malignancy may still be undetected and even undetectable. Nerve conduction studies are normal, but there is mild denervation of muscles in the periphery of the limbs, suggestive of "dying-back neuropathy."

9.2.6 Avitaminosis

The same considerations as given for burning feet syndrome apply to avitaminosis as a cause of restless legs. Unfortunately, vitamin deficiency is not easily demonstrated. In some cases diagnosis can be made only on the basis of substitution therapy.

9.2.7 Psychogenic (Unknown) Etiology

Finally, as mentioned above, very many cases of restless legs syndrome remain unexplained. One cannot help assuming a psychogenic origin in these cases. As in other somatic manifestations of psychological conflict or unbalance, the patients are not susceptible to psychotherapy. Therefore, electrotherapy and other psychologically impressive kinds of therapy are advised.

10 Cerebellar Ataxia

Cerebellar ataxia is a disorder of efferent motor control, and is thus not dependent on the influence of sensory afference. In terms of the neurologic examination, cerebellar ataxia is present not only when closure of the eyes deprives the motor system of visual input compensating for defective proprioceptive information. Rather, equilibrium of the trunk and movements of the limbs are ataxic also when the eyes are open, and visual information on the outside world and on the position of the body is available. According to the localization within the cerebellum (or the cerebellipetal and/or cerebellifugal pathways) there is trunk ataxia, locomotor ataxia, intention tremor, nystagmus, and cerebellar dysarthria. The reader is referred to textbooks for details.

10.1 Multiple Sclerosis

The condition most frequently associated with cerebellar ataxia is multiple sclerosis. The notorious triad described by Charcot, i.e., nystagmus, intention tremor, and cerebellar dysarthria is obviously seen only in rather advanced stages of the disease. This is easily understood when one considers that Charcot had to draw his neurologic experience to a large extent from the inhabitants of a Paris asylum. At the other end of the range, there are children who present with an acute syndrome in which the elements of Charcot's triad are present, but which also includes various signs of brain stem disease, e.g., horizontal gaze paralysis, signs indicative of affection of the long descending motor and ascending sensory pathways, e.g., plantar extensor responses, and sensory impairment of the limbs. There may be paralysis of cranial nerves, diminution of wakefulness, and even respiratory problems. This syndrome was termed in the old literature "encephalitis pontis et cerebelli," and more often than not it has a fatal outcome, or at least it leaves the child seriously disabled.

The majority of cases, of course, fall between these extremes. Suffice it to say here that the firm diagnosis of multiple sclerosis requires multiplicity in space, i.e., signs and symptoms that cannot be attributed to one locus of lesion within the CNS, and also multiplicity in time, i.e., bouts followed by remission. Characteristic combinations of signs and symptoms are: Optic neuritis presenting as monocular or binocular reading problems or global blurring of vision and leading to temporal atrophy of the optic disc; distal numbness and pinprick sensations in the limbs; Lhermitte's sign, i.e., pinprick sensations running down the back or spreading over both shoulders when the head is moved briskly forward; diminution of cutaneous abdominal reflexes; pyramidal tract signs; and bladder dysfunction. A frequent but ill-explained symptom is general fatigability, which is seen in chronic patients.

There are purely chronic cases, though, and here additional examinations are most useful. Among these are the demonstration of multilocular lesions by a battery of evoked potential studies [visual evoked, somatosensory, and brainstem auditory evoked potentials (VEP, SSEP, BAEP)] and by the blink reflex. Neuroimaging may show areas of hypodensity that do not correspond to vascular territories. A frequent yet unspecific neuroimaging finding is global reduction of cerebral volume. Also, CSF study will support the diagnosis by showing IgG synthesis within the CNS by an elevation of the Delpech-Lichtblau quotient: $\dfrac{\text{IgG(CSF)}}{\text{IgG(serum)}} : \dfrac{\text{Alb(CSF)}}{\text{Alb(serum)}}$ and by the demonstration of oligoclonal subfractions of IgG by isoelectric focussing. (Alb, albumin.)

10.2 Postinfectious Encephalomyelitis Affecting the Cerebellum

On the occasion of the first bout, of course, the major differential diagnosis is postinfectious encephalomyelitis. This is an immunologic reaction to viral infection or vaccination. Pathoanatomically, there are multiple foci of perivenous cellular reaction and demyelination, and thus signs and symptoms fulfill the requirement of multiplicity in space. The cerebellum is particularly affected in morbilli and chickenpox. However, no local IgG production in the CSF can be demonstrated. Confirmation of viral infection by serological tests is unfortunately lacking in most cases, because there are many times more viruses than there are tests to demonstrate their presence in the organism.

10.3 Chronic Intoxication

Many instances of chronic intoxication produce Charcot's triad (see Sect 10.1). In addition, reactivity is diminished, because the drugs have a sedative effect. There are no bouts and remissions; at best the condition takes a somewhat fluctuating course. Demonstration of intoxication by means of EEG, toxicologic examination of blood and urine, and kits for antiepileptic drugs are described in Chapt. 26. Discontinuation of intake of the drug in hospital leads either to rapid amelioration or to withdrawal seizures, both of which are of great diagnostic value.

10.4 Infarction in the Territory of the Cerebellar Arteries

In patients of advanced age, acute onset of cerebellar ataxia is seen after embolic or autochthonous occlusion of one of the cerebellar arteries. Sudden onset, lack of headache prior to the event, normal optic discs, and preserved consciousness during the first few day(s) are diagnostic, and CW Ultrasound studies may show a high resistance profile over one of the vertebral arteries. CSF is normal if one decides in favor of a lumbar tap, which, in my view, does not have high priority. Neuroimaging will show cerebellar hypodensity on the 2nd day, and will also show cerebellar hemorrhage which cannot be diagnosed by clinical means alone. In both instances there may be hydrocephalus due to compression of the aqueduct of Sylvius. Recognition of the space-occupying nature of the lesion is vital, because tumors and hemorrhages, and also large infarctions, may threaten the patient by cerebellar herniation interfering with brain stem functions. In these cases ventricular shunting or operative decompression of the posterior fossa is required.

10.5 Late-Onset Cerebellar Atrophy

Predominantly the anterior lobe is affected by late-onset cerebellar atrophy, producing locomotor ataxia, particularly of the legs, and trunk ataxia. The finger-nose maneuver is much less impaired, speech is hardly affected, and there is little or no nystagmus. "Late-onset" refers to the patient's age, and does not infer that all cases have a chronic evolution. There are patients who develop the full-blown syndrome within a day and who are virtually unable to sit or walk. The most frequent cause is chronic alcohol abuse. There are also paraneoplastic cases on record, especially with carcinoma of the ovaries. In some patients no underlying illness or pathologic condition is recognized.

10.6 Space-Occupying Lesion of the Cerebellum or Brain Stem

Tumors or abscesses (or hemorrhage, see Sect. 10.4) located in the cerebellum are more recognizable by headache, tilting of the head toward the side of the lesion ("vestibular tilt"), and neck stiffness than by ataxia. The reason is that these patients do not move freely because they are constantly on the verge of obstruction of the outflow of CSF, which critically worsens their condition. With rare exceptions (angioblastoma or Lindau's tumor, acute hemorrhage) there will be prominence of the optic discs. Diagnosis is made by neuroimaging and/or angiography. A lumbar tap may threaten the patient's life, because lowering of spinal CSF pressure relative to intracranial CSF pressure may lead to herniation of the brain stem into the foramen magnum.

10.7 Miller-Fisher's Syndrome

The variant of Guillain-Barré syndrome accompanied by ophthalmoplegia and cerebellar ataxia, Miller-Fisher's syndrome, is described extensively in Chap. 20. It should be mentioned here that in the early stage the signs of polyneuropathy are limited to attenuation of the proprioceptive reflexes, and ophthalmoplegia may (still) be absent.

10.8 Hereditary Ataxia

The adult variant of hereditary ataxia, originally described by Nonne and Pierre Marie, is characterized by chronic evolution of overall cerebellar ataxia. This means that these patients have serious problems of stance and gait, locomotor ataxia of the upper limbs, and that their speech is quite uncoordinated in all its elements. Phonation varies greatly in volume and in general is loud and crude ("lion's voice"), articulation is blurred, and the patient places stress on virtually every syllable. Nystagmus is conspicuously absent. Often, family history is unremarkable. CSF is normal, and neuroimaging need not necessarily demonstrate cerebellar atrophy, at least not in the first stage of the disease. There are no bouts or remissions, and the course is relentlessly progressive. Eventually, the patients present with pyramidal signs. Atrophy of the optic nerve may also occur.

10.9 Olivopontocerebellar Atrophy

A similar condition is olivopontocerebellar atrophy, although this runs a much faster course. Usually, it begins with extrapyramidal symptoms reminiscent of the akinetic variant of Parkinson's disease, which are followed by cerebellar ataxia. Slowly but surely progressive dementia appears. Brain stem signs may include horizontal gaze paralysis.

10.10 Combined Degeneration of the Spinal Cord

The syndrome of combined degeneration of the spinal cord will be described in Chap. 29. Here it may suffice to mention that ataxia may be a prominent sign in this disease.

10.11 Wernicke's Encephalopathy (Thiamine Deficiency)

Also, Wernicke's encephalopathy owing to thiamine deficiency has been discussed elsewhere (Chap. 6). The prominent features are cerebellar ataxia, oculomotor and pupillomotor disturbances, and, less frequently, attenuation of vigilance. Nystagmus, ataxia, oculomotor and pupillo-motor disturbances combined with mental alteration in the patient should arouse suspicion of this treatable disease.

10.12 Tabes Dorsalis and Sensory Polyneuropathy

Spinal or sensory ataxia is one consequence of tabes dorsalis. In contrast to cerebellar ataxia, the motor incoordination in these cases is due to impairment of sensory input from the limbs, which can be at least partially compensated for by visual control (for the diagnosis of tabes dorsalis, see Chap. 29). The same holds true for certain cases of sensory polyneuropathy, which are diagnosed by distal paresthesia, attenuation of proprioceptive reflexes, and slowing of nerve conduction.

10.13 Creutzfeldt-Jakob Disease, Cerebellar Form

There is an ataxic variant of Creutzfeld-Jakob disease. Diagnosis is almost impossible in vivo. EEG does not necessarily show the characteristic triphasic complexes, neuroimaging alterations are unspecific, and CSF findings are normal. The diagnosis can be made only by considering the particularly rapid progression of the syndrome, which is eventually enriched by signs of affection of other motor systems, e.g., pyramidal tract and basal ganglia.

11 Choreic Syndrome

Hyperkinesia of the choreic type is not easily differentiated from psychogenic hyperkinesia, because the involuntary movements are more coordinated than tremor or myoclonus. They involve parts as well as groups of muscles, and the resulting movements may have a resemblance to expressive gestures or grimacing. This is true of all variants and all ages.

11.1 Sydenham's Chorea

An inflammatory disease of the basal ganglia which may accompany rheumatic heart disease in childhood, Sydenham's chorea is invariably assumed to be psychogenic in its initial stage. The young patients are therefore disciplined for misbehavior in school or at the table, rather than being presented to the doctor. If they are, the diagnosis is not easily arrived at. In general, emotional instability is part of the disease. The characteristic hypotonicity of limb muscles is hard to recognize, because few doctors are experienced enough to judge a child's muscle tone. Useful signs are:

- Chameleon's tongue, i.e., the inability to keep the protruded tongue stretched out of the mouth for a period of, say, 10 s. The reason is involuntary retraction of the tongue, a symptom of orofacial hyperkinesia.
- Gordon's knee phenomenon. After eliciting the patellar jerk from the child sitting on a chair or on the bedside, the leg does not fall down in a phasic movement, but rather the contraction of the quadriceps femoris muscle is released slowly, in a tonic way.

For examination, it is useful if the patient lies barefoot in a supine position. Frequently, one will discover slight choreic movements of the toes which are not normally seen in psychogenic hyperkinesia, because they have no expressive function. Medical examination reveals cardiac signs, mostly disease of the mitral valve, in roughly 30% of cases, and alteration of various laboratory parameters, indicating an acute inflammatory process mostly of a rheumatic nature.

11.2 Chorea Gravidarum

A very similar syndrome occurs in rare instances in advanced pregnancy. A high proportion of these patients have been suffering from Sydenham's chorea in infancy. Many have had rheumatic heart disease. The condition is rather benign and should not prompt interruption of pregnancy. It ceases after childbirth.

11.3 Huntington's Disease

A very familial condition is Huntington's disease, yet rarely does the patient admit that other members of the family are affected. Usually, the hyperkinesia begins in distal muscles, and again, examination of barefooted patients is very revealing. Only at a later stage are proximal muscles affected. Invariably, signs of "choreophrenia", which is a blend of dementia and behavioral abnormalities, develop (Chap. 12.7). Muscle tone is very likely to be increased (rigidity), and the chameleon's tongue sign is present.

There is a variant of Huntington's chorea where the movements are for a long period of time confined to the orofacial muscles. These patients develop an extrapyramidal type of dysarthria with blurred, monotonous speech, and grimacing. Quite frequently, the involuntary movements of the tongue and the incoordination of oral, pharyngeal, and laryngeal muscles make chewing and swallowing impossible. This should prevent a misdiagnosis of psychogenic hyperkinesia.

11.4 Hypersensitivity to Dopaminergic Drugs

The choreic movements after long-term *levodopa therapy* or therapy with dopamine agonists in patients with Parkinson's disease are too well known to require detailed discussion here. The movements particularly affect the muscles of the shoulder girdle and the muscles which move the head, earlier than they affect the distal hand and foot muscles. Strangely enough, many patients with Parkinson's disease are ready to tolerate this hyperkinesia although it is a great social handicap, because they are satisfied with the motor effect of levodopa. The doctor, however, should not continue with the same dosage in these cases.

43

11.5 Hypersensitivity to Neuroleptic Drugs

In the adult the most frequent cause of choreic hyperkinesia is currently intake of drugs acting on the basal ganglia. These may range from antivertiginous drugs, which cause acute chorea in case of hypersensitivity (which is very common), to neuroleptic drugs, which are prescribed with regrettable frequency as "minor tranquilizers." The acute drug-induced chorea responds so favorably to intravenously administered anticholinergic substances that this effect is diagnostic.

11.6 Tardive Dyskinesia Following Years of Neuroleptic Treatment

Much more difficult to treat is tardive dyskinesia following years of neuroleptic treatment. This prolonged treatment alters the characteristics of receptors in the motor system to such a degree that no predictable pharmacologic effect can be achieved. Inquiry about a chronic intake of neuroleptics and/or about a history of psychiatric illness should be routine in the case of choreiform movements of progressive evolution in the adult.

11.7 Arteriosclerotic Chorea

Choreic hyperkinesia is rarely caused by cerebral arteriosclerosis, in marked contrast to parkinsonian symptoms, which are not infrequently seen in the latter condition.

11.8 Other Medical Conditions
(Polycythemia, Paraproteinemia, Cerebral Vasculitis)

Three medical conditions, however, should be considered in patients of middle or advanced age before making the diagnosis of Huntington's chorea. These are *polycythemia*, which is seen in patients presenting with chronic congestion of the lungs with weakness of the left ventricle (cor pulmonale) and very severe *paraproteinemia*. The medical signs and symptoms need not be prominent, but must be locked for.

It should be mentioned in passing that *cerebral vasculitis* of all sorts, especially the variant due to visceral lupus erythematosus, may affect the vessels irrigating the corpus striatum, and thus lead to a choreic syndrome.

11.9 Hepatolenticular Degeneration (Wilson's Disease)

This rare hereditary disorder of copper metabolism usually leads to parkinsonian symptoms and to flapping tremor. Sometimes it presents with a choreic syndrome. One should entertain this diagnosis when a patient exhibits a choreic syndrome between the ages of 15 and 25 years, because it is relatively easily confirmed and leads to therapeutic consequences. Medical findings include hepatomegaly, and low levels of copper and ceruloplasmin, the protein that carries copper in the plasma. Copper excretion in the urine is greatly enhanced, as is the excretion of various amino acids.

The pathognomonic light-brownish Kayser-Fleischer corneal ring is best seen with the slit lamp.

Examination of relatives is strongly indicated.

11.10 Perinatal Brain Damage

Chorea due to perinatal brain damage is easily diagnosed because onset occurs very early in childhood (as opposed to school age in Sydenham's chorea) and brain damage is usually known. In most cases history reveals perinatal jaundice due to Rhesus incompatibility.

11.11 Psychogenic "Chorea"

This condition occurs at all ages and is mostly a diagnosis by exclusion. Some of the distinguishing signs that are conspicuously absent in *psychogenic choreiform hyperkinesia* have already been mentioned. There is no chameleon's tongue, no hypotonicity, no Gordon's knee phenomenon, and the toes are not affected in the beginning of the disorder. Rather, the hyperkinesia affects primarily the facial muscles, arms, and hands. Observing the undressed patient, one will notice that only groups of muscles are involved, whereas twitching of parts of muscles and/or crude fasciculationlike movements, which are invariably present in advanced chorea, are missing, as is "choreophrenia."

The picture may be blurred by the fact that some psychogenic patients also take neuroleptic drugs. In this case, there will be some improvement after intravenous injection of anticholinergic substances. A similar effect, however, may be achieved with saline.

12 Dementia

With the increase in life expectancy, dementia has become a central medical problem. The challenge to the diagnostician is to single out treatable conditions that can be either cured or at least slowed down in their course of progression. The table shows that there is more to dementia than just degenerative or atherosclerotic disease of the brain. The important discussion as to whether the global concept of dementia is still adequate is beyond the scope of this book. Any disease process listed in the table is multifocal rather than diffuse in the trivial sense of the term. Consequently, it appears that the assumption of a unitary "chronic brain syndrome" is unrealistic, in that it ignores the results of many decades of neuropsychological research into the differential organization of cognitive functions in the brain. Accepting the need for precise analysis of the multifaceted syndromes of cognitive disturbance in organic brain disease will open an avenue for neuropsychological therapy, which might, at least in a proportion of cases, complement medical therapy.

12.1 Senile Dementia of the Alzheimer Type (SDAT)

SDAT is considered a degenerative disease with onset in the 6th decade or beyond. It usually starts with difficulty in recalling recent events. Next, there will be impoverishment of vocabulary and syntax without actual aphasia, followed by other neuropsychological disturbances, such as spatial disorientation. There is a striking contrast between the marked neuropsychological impairment and the well-preserved awareness of social behavior. Neurologic findings include akinesia, rigidity, and occasional pyramidal tract signs.

EEG shows slow activity in the low alpha or theta range. Usually there are no focal signs, and neuroimaging may be surprisingly normal.

Dementia definitely cannot be equated with brain atrophy, nor does brain volume correlate with cognitive performance. CSF is normal. Diagnosis rests on the steadily progressive evolution of the syndrome described above, and on exclusion of the conditions listed in the table.

12.2 Subcortical Arteriosclerotic Encephalopathy (Binswanger's Disease)

A vascular disease of the brain, Binswanger's disease, affects mainly the long penetrating arteries supplying the white matter of the hemispheres, basal ganglia, and brain stem in chronically hypertensive patients. The basic evolution is toward dementia, which is due to a complex disconnection process because of progressive demyelination. Social behavior is not so well preserved as in SDAT. In addition to this progressive course there are repeated "little strokes" in the territories mentioned above, which add focal neurologic signs to the syndrome Doppler ultrasound studies show little or no change in the extracranial arteries. EEG is uncharacteristic. Evoked potential studies show signs of deficient transmission of signals. There is no relation between the severity of morphological alteration as seen in neuroimaging and the degree of dementia.

Diagnosis is provided by neuroimaging. There are bilateral areas of hypodensity in the white matter, usually beginning in the neighborhood of the anterior horns of the ventricles, and extending over a period of years across most of the white matter. In addition, there are lacunes as residua of the intermittent strokes.

Medical findings include arterial hypertension and, frequently, elevation of hematocrit, and other signs of derangement of the rheological properties of blood. Prognosis depends on control of these medical parameters.

12.3 Multi-Infarction Dementia

There is certainly a great deal of overlap between Binswanger's disease and multi-infarction dementia. In my view, the latter concept is broader and somewhat diffuse. It was introduced with the view of distinguishing between "degenerative" and "vascular" dementia. The characteristic traits of multi-infarct dementia are strokes in the patient's history and striking neurologic signs in the presence of deterioration of the cognitive processes. Additional findings may be those of large-vessel disease, as detected by CW Ultrasound study, and various kinds of risk factors. However, hypertension is not necessarily present. Neuroimaging shows diminution of hemispheric volume, and lacunar and territorial infarctions, the latter corresponding to the vascular supply of larger vessels.

12.4 Tumor of the Frontal Lobe

A frontal lobe tumor may go undetected for a long time. The patients slowly undergo changes in behavior, lose interest in their usual activities and personal relations, and take less care of themselves. They appear increasingly slow in mentation. Many of them do not complain of headache, or at least not very urgently. Neurologic findings may just show grasping and groping reflexes and a tendency to maintain any position of the limbs imposed on them during examination. Papilledema is not present in all cases. EEG shows slow waves over the frontal lead(s). Neuroimaging permits recognition of the tumor.

12.5 Severe Traumatic Brain Damage

A patient with severe traumatic brain damage may have gross psychopathological and neuropsychological alterations. If one hemisphere is affected there will be neuropsychological impairment such as aphasia, spatial disorientation, and disturbance of attention, of memory, and of the ability to adapt to rapidly changing demands, to name but a few. After brain stem damage there are predominantly emotional changes, and a loss of spontaneity.

The diagnosis poses no problems if the trauma is known or detected by neuroimaging. Traumatic brain stem damage may lead to atrophy of the brain stem and the cerebellum, but this is not so in all cases. EEG is usually normal, but electrophysiological studies may show signs of brain stem damage.

12.6 Dementia in Parkinson's Disease

It is by no means only on islands in the Pacific that dementia occurs in Parkinson's disease. It has been recognized that roughly one-third of parkinsonian patients have moderate to severe cognitive deficit in addition to the incapacitating influence of the motor disorder.

12.7 Huntington's Disease

The well-known hyperkinesia is not the only sign in Huntington's disease: virtually all patients eventually exhibit both personality alteration and cognitive impairment. Personality changes include loosening of social bonds, loss of tact, aggressive behavior, and sexual disinhibition. The psychopathological syndrome may precede the extrapyramidal syndrome (see als Chap. 11). If there is no family history available, tentative diagnosis may be Pick's disease or general paresis of the insane (see Sect. 12.10).

12.8 Communicating Hydrocephalus

It is an imbalance between production and absorption of CSF that causes communicating hydrocephalus. The condition may follow disease of the meninges, such as subarachnoid hemorrhage (SAH) or meningitis, or may occur with no recognizable cause. Signs and symptoms are rather characteristic, and permit distinction from other forms of dementia. The first presenting sign is loss of spontaneity and flattening of affect. This indifference is followed by a peculiar disturbance of gait, erroneously called gait apraxia. The patients walk about with small, hesitating steps, hardly lifting their feet from the ground. They resist any attempt to accelerate their walking tempo; if pulled by the outstretched arms they will lean backward. In an advanced stage they no longer leave their bed, and if one tries to lift them up the whole body stiffens in resistance. Finally, they succumb to urinary incontinence. At this stage at the latest, neuroimaging study is indicated, but should preferably be done earlier, before irreversible brain damage has occurred. The typical finding is enlargement of the ventricles, in particular of the temporal horns, while the pattern of gyri and sulci is hardly recognizable. Radioactive substances brought into the subarachnoid space penetrate into the ventricles, which they normally do not.

12.9 Alcohol Abuse

It is only for the sake of comprehensiveness that a brief mention is made here of alcohol abuse. The diagnosis of dementia owing to chronic alcoholism should pose no problem. Rapid deterioration of cognitive performance in an alcoholic patient should arouse suspicion of *bilateral subdural hematoma*, which is easily recognized by neuroimaging.

12.10 General Paresis of the Insane

Although it has become rare, general paresis of the insane has not been completely eliminated. Textbooks of psychiatry describe a spectrum of psychopathologic alterations ranging from expansive, euphoric behavior to aspontaneous dementia. Usually there are the personality changes described above for Huntington's disease. The widespread syphilitic disease of the brain also affects areas that have motor functions, such as the frontoparietal area of the cortex, basal ganglia, and cerebellum. Consequently, all kinds of fine motor functions are grossly impaired. Since speaking is a motor function that requires particularly precise alternation of innervation patterns, dysarthria is invariably present. There are all kinds of pupillary alterations, ranging from Argyll

Robertson pupil (see Chap. 29) to unequally dilated, nonreactive pupils. Frequently, there is tabetic affection of the spinal cord with loss of ankle and knee jerks (see Chap. 29).

Blood tests demonstrate activity of the syphilitic process. CSF shows moderate pleocytosis, elevation of protein levels, and, in particular, of IgG. Of course, reactions for syphilis are strongly positive.

12.11 Pick's Disease

A systemic atrophy, Pick's disease involves either the frontal or the temporal lobe of the brain. The frontal variant is much more common; it is characterized by the personality alterations described for Huntington's disease, while cognitive impairment is relatively sparse. Neurologic signs are less prominent than in SDAT. In the variant affecting the temporal lobe there may be aphasia that cannot be classified along the lines of the well-known aphasic syndromes of vascular origin. Diagnosis is made by neuroimaging and exclusion of general paresis of the insane.

12.12 Psychogenic Pseudodementia

There are two variants of psychogenic pseudodementia. One is completely hysterical and has an abrupt onset, which facilitates diagnosis. The patients appear devoid of affect and aspontaneous, and hardly react to their surroundings. If interviewed, their answers are grossly inappropriate. They are likely to pretend they are completely disoriented with regard to time, place, and person; the latter feature being rarely seen in organic disease. If questioned further, they frequently give answers that are only slightly off-target. For example, in May they will give June or April as the month of the year, and they will pretend to be unable to guess the profession of the doctor, in spite of his white coat and the "medical surroundings." The overall impression is that of reluctance, hesitancy, and rather infantile behavior. Neurologic examination is very useful in these cases, because the patients pretend not to understand even fairly simple commands.

Another variant that is not so easily recognized is seen in patients who do have organic brain disease and whose cognitive performance is, in fact, somewhat impaired. Yet for some reason they strongly exaggerate their impairment. This condition is frequently seen in patients seeking compensation for brain injury suffered in an accident. It might be necessary to apply elaborate psychological testing procedures to be able to demonstrate that the patients' performance is more or less random, because they do not distinguish between easy and difficult tasks.

13 Facial "Hyperkinesia" (Involuntary Movements of Facial Musculature)

When a patient presents with involuntary movements of the facial musculature, the first question is: is the problem of organic or psychic origin? Unilateral hyperkinesia is always organic, but the bilateral variety may be psychic.

Unilateral movements have either a peripheral or a central origin. Peripheral movements, of course, are mediated by the seventh nerve and are therefore limited to muscles innervated by this nerve. In other words: if there is hyperkinesia not only of the facial muscles proper, but also of, for example, the masticatory muscles and/or the tongue, a central origin has to be assumed.

13.1 Associated Movements After Seventh Nerve Palsy

The most frequent type of unilateral movements are associated movements during, and after incomplete, recovery from seventh nerve palsy. In these cases, the hyperkinesia plays upon a state of either residual weakness or tonic increase of facial innervation. In other words: the two halves of the face do not look alike even when completely at rest. The lids are either wider apart or closer together on the side of the hyperkinesia, and the nasolabial fold is either softer or more pronounced. The associated movements occur during spontaneous eyeblinks, while the patient speaks, or during any alteration in facial expression. The hyperkinesia can be seen, for example, in closure of the eyelids, while the patient moves his mouth, or lifts the corner of his mouth upon a movement of the upper face. History will reveal that there has been complete facial paralysis. The phenomenon is due to "cross talk" (transmission of excitation between neighboring nerve fibers) within the incompletely recovered facial nerve.

13.2 Hemifacial Spasm

The occurrence of hemifacial spasm is spontaneous, that is it occurs at rest, but it increases in amplitude and frequency upon any facial innervation or emotional movement, both of which, of course, frequently go together. It consists of irregular "tonic-clonic" synchronous movements of the entire facial musculature of one side, including the platysma. Tonic-clonic means that there are both contractions that last several seconds and rapid contractions at a frequency of 3–5/s. The picture resembles the effect of electrical stimulation of the main branch of the facial nerve at the mandibular angle if applied with varying duration and at varying intervals.

It is assumed that there is a partial lesion in the peripheral course of the facial nerve, which produces volleys of impulses travelling in virtually all of the nerve fibers. This concept would explain why in some cases there is at the same time some degree of peripheral facial weakness.

13.3 Hemifacial Myokymia

The synchronous contractions of hemifacial spasm should not be confounded with the showers of very delicate movements that run over various parts of the facial musculature in hemifacial myokymia, again strictly unilateral. In contrast to the two conditions described above, there is no gross motor effect. The picture somehow resembles the fasciculations seen in motor neuron disease, but it occurs in a completely different setting. In fact, this hemifacial myokymia is quite strongly suggestive of multiple sclerosis.

13.4 Epilepsia Partialis Continua

Rapid clonic, very rarely tonic-clonic, unilateral contractions restricted to one area of the facial musculature, sometimes limited to an area as small as the triangular muscle, and which last for hours or days, are termed epilepsia partialis continua, a term which is self-explanatory, or Koshevnikoff's epilepsy. The problem of the underlying cause, as well as EEG findings, is discussed in Chap. 38.

13.5 Drug-Induced Hyperkinesia

Bilateral movements of the facial musculature frequently convey the impression that they reflect the patient's affective state, but are psychogenic only in a minority of instances; currently, the most frequent cause is drug-induced hyperkinesia. The movements are not confined to muscles innervated by the seventh nerve. In the face, in addition to lifting of the eyebrows or closing of the eyes, there is opening and closing of the mouth, lateral movements of the jaws, and/or protrusion or bizarre rolling of the tongue. Frequently, neck and shoulder muscles are also involved in all kinds of twisting movements. This type of hyperkinesia is most common after long-term treatment of Parkinson's disease with dopaminergic drugs. In this case diagnosis is easy. Patients who have undergone long-term neuroleptic treatment for psychiatric conditions may exhibit the same symptoms, but are not likely to report the circumstances to a doctor they do not know well.

Finally, there are patients who are hypersensitive to neuroleptics and display the full syndrome described above after ingestion of very few, sometimes just one dose of a neuroleptic drug which they took simply to calm themselves or to avoid motion sickness. In contrast to the first variants, this is an acute event. In these cases, intravenous injection of an anticholinergic substance immediately resolves the hyperkinesia and permits diagnosis. Unfortunately, the chronic hyperkinesias are due to severe alteration of receptor characteristics and are therefore not easily treated, if they are susceptible to treatment at all.

13.6 Choreic Hyperkinesia

Three conditions involve choreic hyperkinesia: Sydenham's chorea, Huntington's chorea, and chorea gravidarum. They are discussed in Chap. 11. Here it is important to note that choreic facial movements are eminently expressive in nature, to the extent that very frequently they are taken to be psychogenic. There is, in fact, no distinctive feature in the movements themselves, at least not in the initial stage. Additional symptoms can be of help. Among these are the sign of the "chameleon's tongue," the inability of the patient to keep his tongue protruded because of constant interference by involuntary movements. Furthermore, there may be hypotonicity of limb muscles, which, however, requires some experience to judge, and "Gordon's knee phenomenon," i.e., a delay of several seconds in the relaxation of the quadriceps femoris muscle after the patellar jerk has been elicited. As a result, the outstretched calf does not fall back abruptly, but returns very slowly to the original position. Frequently, choreic movements can be seen in the fingers and toes in an early stage of the diseases.

13.7 Psychogenic Facial Tic

All these additional symptoms are absent in psychogenic facial tic. Movements are very rapid, always bilateral, but not always synchronous. They vary in frequency and intensity and are most pronounced in the upper face, sometimes assuming the form of tonic-clonic lid closure, which unfortunately may be the first sign of extrapyramidal disease. Diagnosis is extremely difficult and is frequently accomplished only after follow-up of weeks or even months. It is understood that the effect of treatment gives no definite diagnostic clue. Errors are possible both ways: psychogenic tic may temporarily respond favorably to anticholinergic treatment, while organic disease may be resistant to the drugs chosen.

14 First Epileptic Seizure(s) in Adulthood

As a rule of thumb, epileptic seizures of all sorts occurring in infancy and childhood most probably indicate what is loosely (and for want of a more precise explanation) called idiopathic epilepsy. A first seizure in adult age should give rise to a thorough search for organic, toxic, or metabolic brain disease or an extracerebral condition that might lead to seizures. The main weakness of this rule of thumb is that even in infancy, and even when hereditary influence is possibly operative, the cause of the epilepsy might be an organic brain lesion, e.g., an arteriovenous malformation or perinatal brain damage. Epilepsy is a multifactorial condition. We suggest therefore that any epileptic patient should have neuroimaging examination with contrast at least once in his life, and the earlier the better. Neuroimaging is particularly essential in cases of focal seizures, or when there is a change in the type of seizure.

When the first seizure occurs in adult age, the conditions listed in the table should be considered very seriously, which implies repeat examination of the patient, should the first series of tests be unrevealing. For the sake of brevity we are going to speak of seizures of the grand mal type, but most of what is being said in this chapter applies also to partial or complex partial seizures.

A preliminary problem is, of course, to establish whether the seizure really was epileptic in nature. Unfortunately, more often than not there is no eye witness, or the description given is not very helpful because the observer was too excited to record the relevant details. As discussed in Chap. 31, valuable signs like a bitten tongue or lip, enuresis, or elevated level of serum creatine kinase are often lacking, and the EEG may show merely an unspecific abnormality.

In case of doubt it is wise to assume that the patient has in fact had an epileptic seizure, and to proceed with a search for the underlying cause.

14.1 Withdrawal Syndrome (Alcohol or Drugs)

By far the most frequent causes are abuse of alcohol or tranquilizing drugs, and brain tumor or abscess.

Toxic seizures are, as a rule, withdrawal seizures, and their appearance indicates that there has been a regular intake of large doses over a prolonged period of time. Just what constitutes a large dose in the individual case varies greatly. This is one of the many reasons why the history quite frequently remains obscure, particularly since regular intake is to a surprising extent considered socially acceptable and hence not worth reporting to the doctor, who therefore has to rely more on personal observation.

A most valuable sign is a fine tremor of the outstretched fingers and hands. Many patients will report that the tremor has an increased amplitude (not frequency) in the morning, that is, after overnight abstinence, and wanes during the day, that is, under the effect of alcohol or drug intake. Familial or "essential" tremor also diminishes following alcohol consumption, but the tremor excursions are coarser, and the condition usually starts in late childhood. EEG is usually normal. Neuroimaging will show a global reduction of hemispheric volume, and usually also cerebellar "atrophy." The inverted commas suggest that the diminution of volume indicates dystrophy rather than atrophy and is reversible in some patients, provided they abstain from drinking.

Withdrawal seizures may herald a tremulous state which will develop during the next 1–3 days, and this condition is potentially fatal if medical treatment in the intensive care unit is not given early enough. Withdrawal from drugs is much more difficult to recognize both by history and by medical examination, and treatment will moreover, be prolonged, requiring the full armamentarium of intensive care.

14.2 Brain Tumor

The next consideration is brain tumor, and since seizures occur mainly in histologically benign, slow-growing gliomas or in vascular malformations, history may be of little help, as is, in many cases, routine neurologic examination. Neuroimaging with contrast is the first choice among the ancillary examinations, and it should be repeated if the study is normal and no other cause is found.

14.3 Brain Abscess

An abscess of the brain will not escape detection by neuroimaging. Laboratory findings need not be suggestive of inflammatory disease. EEG, as a rule, shows focal abnormality in the very slow delta range, plus general alteration. Thorough ear, nose, and throat (ENT) examination and chest X-ray are minimal requirements.

14.4 Brain Trauma

Following brain trauma, epilepsy may appear with a latency of years, so that the patient often forgets reporting the event. History taking is of particular importance in these cases.

14.5 Viral Encephalitis

Any viral encephalitis may start with epileptic seizures. The triad of epileptic fits, generalized slowing and irregularity of the EEG, and disorientation or frankly psychotic behavior is most suggestive. CSF may contain an increased number of lymphocytic cells, while protein and lactate levels are normal or only slightly increased (the lactate level rises when bacteria reduce glucose). A rare but most dangerous condition is *herpes simplex encephalitis*. It usually starts with a series of epileptic fits, which are followed by clouding of consciousness, hemiplegia, and aphasia, if the left temporal lobe is affected. The patient's condition rapidly deteriorates to coma and decerebrate rigidity owing to massive swelling of the temporal lobes, which thus exert pressure on the brain stem. In the neuroimaging study there is hypodensity of limbic areas of the temporal and later also of the frontal lobes, which evolves over the 1st week. During the first few days, the EEG shows unspecific abnormality. The appearance of periodic high-voltage, slow-amplitude complexes over both temporal leads is highly suggestive of the diagnosis. CSF routine examination reveals moderate lymphocytic pleocytosis and an increase in the protein level. The presence of herpes simplex virus can be demonstrated in CSF directly and by ELISA technique.

14.6 Arteriovenous Malformation

An arteriovenous malformation can be suspected when neuroimaging study with contrast shows a circumscribed irregular area of hyperdensity in the convexity of one hemisphere with no surrounding edema. This diagnosis is confirmed by angiography.

14.7 Thrombosis of the Cerebral Sinus(es)

Epileptic seizures may follow thrombosis of the cerebral sinuses, because there is hypoxia of, and diapedesis bleeding into, the area of the hemisphere(s) where the drainage is blocked. Vigilance is, as a rule, decreased before focal signs are demonstrable. The same holds true for the EEG, where generalized slowing prevails. The radiological signs are described in Chap. 26.

14.8 Carcinomatous Meningitis

Headache and mild neck stiffness necessitates a lumbar tap. Carcinomatous meningitis should be suspected if there is a small increase in atypical cells (which have to be identified by cytologic examination) considerable increase in the protein level, and a decrease in the glucose level in the CSF, glucose being metabolized by tumor cells.

14.9 Metabolic Encephalopathy

The medical consultant usually diagnoses metabolic encephalopathy on the basis of characteristic patterns of laboratory findings, which cannot be described here in detail.

14.10 Multiple Sclerosis

It should be mentioned in passing that in (very) rare instances multiple sclerosis may start with epileptic seizures, generalized as well as partial.

14.11 Extracerebral Disease, e.g., Cardiac Conditions, Hypoglycemia

Epileptic fits are not infrequently caused by intermittent interference with the oxygen supply to the brain, owing to a cardiac condition. Recurrent asystolia, i.e., Adams-Stokes disease, is the best-known example, but there are other conditions that make thorough cardiological examination advisable, especially in elderly patients. Hypoglycemia as a cause of epileptic seizures is discussed in Chap. 38.

15 Footdrop, Bilateral

In contrast to unilateral footdrop, which may be of central or peripheral origin, flaccid bilateral footdrop always indicates disease of the peripheral nerves or of the muscles. Onset may be insidious to the extent that the patient gradually gets used to the alteration of gait and is hardly aware that it is a sign of disease, or it may be acute and therefore alarming.

15.1. Chronic

15.1.1 Polyneuropathy. Chronic development of footdrop is seen in polyneuropathy, especially of metabolic origin, including diabetes, or of toxic origin, including alcohol. The diagnosis is discussed at length in Chap. 34 on symmetrical areflexia.

15.1.2 Charcot-Marie-Tooth Disease. The same holds true for the second important disease state to be considered, namely, hereditory motor sensory neuropathy (HMSN), and, in particular, Charcot-Marie-Tooth disease (for details see Chap. 34).

15.1.3 Dystrophia Myotonica (Steinert's Disease). Particularly protracted is the development of the footdrop in a degenerative muscular disease which was described by Curschmann and Steinert and which is termed dystrophia myotonica, or Steinert's disease. The name implies that there are two components, one dystrophic and the other myotonic in nature. The clinical picture is most characteristic. The peculiar gait of these patients is striking. The severe paresis or paralysis of the extensor muscles acting on the foot is a particular hindrance when the patient attempts to turn round. He cannot do this by rotating the body on one heel as normals do, because this requires lifting of the forefoot, which is impossible for these patients. Instead, he turns round slowly, in small steps, always lifting the knees excessively in order to overcome the footdrop.

Upon inspection one is struck by the flaccid posture and poor musculature of these patients. Men usually are bald, and women have very thin hair. The face is lean and expressionless (facies myopathica/ myopathic face). On close examination one may not be able to visualize the retina by funduscopy because of cataract of the lens. The dystrophic process affects particularly the following muscles, which are likely to be virtually absent: the sternomastoid and brachioradial muscles, and the extensors and pronators of the foot. However, there is widespread dystrophy, which affects virtually all muscles of the face, trunk, and limbs. Reflexes are diminished or absent because the muscles do not respond sufficiently to the afferent nervous volley. An EMG shows a myopathic pattern.

The myotonic component is sometimes present in the patient who complains that he cannot voluntarily loosen his grip immediately. Examination reveals a delay in relaxation after forceful innervation which, again, is most conveniently tested in the patient's grip. "Percussion myotonia" can also be elicited by a brisk blow with the acute side of the reflex hammer on the patient's thenar or on the outstretched tongue placed upon a spatula. The reaction consists of a prolonged contraction which relaxes only over a period of roughly three seconds. The myotonic reaction is very clearly recognizable by EMG, when the insertion or any movement of the needle is followed by a train of action potentials.

15.2 Acute

15.2.1 Medial Herniation of a Lumbar Disc. In acute bilateral footdrop the diagnostic decision must be swift and efficient, because there may be a need for immediate surgical intervention. This is the case when the cause of the extensor muscle paralysis is a medial – as opposed to dorsolateral – herniation of a lumbar disc.

The patient may complain of lumbar pain with irradiation to the flexor aspect of both legs, and may have lumbar stiffness due to reflex contraction of the trunk muscles. Ankle jerks are diminished or absent, and there is bilateral Lasègue's sign. Micturition is usually blocked, and sensory impairment, i.e., numbness and decreased awareness of touch and painful stimuli, will rapidly spread from the feet to cover both legs. CT myelography (see Chap. 60) must be performed at once, because there is virtually no therapeutic alternative to surgery, and the only question is the level of herniation.

15.2.2 Polyneuropathy. Only in very rare instances does polyneuropathy lead to micturition impairment. It certainly does not lead to severe lumbar pain or lumbar stiffness. Electroneurography is of no diagnostic help during the first few days of the disease. In case of doubt one should consider which error would have more serious consequences for the patient. In my view, it is less hazardous to perform myelography on a patient with polyneuropathy than to miss the diagnosis of a herniated disk. If the pressure on the fibers of the cauda equina is not relieved immediately, a delayed operation will be followed by only partial recovery or no recovery at all.

16 Footdrop, Unilateral

The condition may be of peripheral or central origin, and under each of these circumstances a variety of causes should be considered. The basic question, peripheral vs central, is not always easy to decide. More than one patient has received conservative or even operative treatment for a slipped disk, while in fact suffering either from cortical monoparesis due to ischemic stroke, or from a crossed leg palsy (see below).

The following signs help to distinguish between central and peripheral footdrop:

- Circumduction of the leg, which is due to enhanced extensor tone, indicates central paresis, and is observable when the patient enters the consultation room. Exaggerated elevation of the foot points to a peripheral paresis.
- The presence of associated movements in the entire leg upon attempting to perform fine movements of the toes, or of discrete rotatory movements in the ankle jerk, is characteristic of central motor disorder. Absence of the required movement is seen in peripheral paresis.
- The level of reflexes: an enhanced ankle jerk reveals a lesion in the central motor pathways, and a diminished or absent jerk indicates a disturbance of conduction in the peripheral reflex arc. Equal ankle jerks are equivocal: when a lesion affects the peroneal nerve or is confined to the L-5 root, one must not expect reflex changes. The plantar extensor response may be absent or equivocal in central footdrop.

More difficult to evaluate are:

- Muscle tone, which is often unremarkable and does not correspond

to the expected pattern: enhanced equals central; diminished equals peripheral.
- Muscular atrophy, which is not to be expected in *acute* footdrop.
- Distribution of sensory disturbance, if present. A rule of thumb is that *unilateral* stocking distribution is more suggestive of a central lesion, in contrast to the well-known peripheral and segmental distribution. If the anatomy of sensory innervation is not familiar to the examiner, he should draw a sketch and compare it to the schemata in the books.

Of course, electromyography and conduction velocity studies are extremely helpful. However, in most instances the decision can be arrived at without ancillary examination.

16.1 Peripheral

Once the peripheral origin is established, the locus of lesion can be assessed tentatively: is this a case of isolated drop of the foot and toes, or is there weakness in other muscles? If so, is it limited to the supply of the peroneal nerve, or does it extend to the tibial nerve? Affection of muscles innervated by one lumbar root or two neighboring roots can be diagnosed prior to EMG, but this requires careful examination and anatomical knowledge. Finally, assessment of the onset – acute or insidious – is very helpful (see below).

The differential diagnosis embraces the following conditions:

Compression Neuropathy

16.1.1 (Crossed Legs Palsy). This is a compression neuropathy of the peroneal nerve, including the superficial and deep branches, which is accompanied by sensory symptoms, such as pinprick paresthesias and hypesthesia. Although the cause is repeated pressure on the peroneal nerve just below the knee in persons who have the habit of crossing their legs while sitting, the onset of weakness is usually acute. Careful history taking is essential. Nerve conduction studies confirm the diagnosis by demonstrating a block of conduction at the place of damage.

There are patients who are liable to pressure paralysis, and this condition may be familial. One should ask for similar instances of acute, transient weakness, e.g., of the ulnar nerve. One should not ignore the family history, and conduction study should be extended to other nerves with a view to demonstrating general slowing of conduction in these admittedly rare cases. If possible, relatives of the patient should also be examined.

63

16.1.2 Inflammatory or Neoplastic Lesions of the Lateral Calf and Baker's Cyst of the Knee Joint. The peroneal nerve may be be damaged by inflammatory or neoplastic lesions in the lateral calf. *Neuroma* or a Baker's cyst of the knee joint are other rare causes of damage to this nerve. The first diagnostic step is to establish the locus of lesion close to the head of the fibula by neurologic examination and recording of nerve conduction. Radiological and sonographic examination are usually mandatory, but these ancillary examinations can be correctly focussed only when clinical localization is provided.

16.1.3 Traumatic Lesion of the Peroneal Nerve. Any kind of *injury to the knee* or proximal fracture of the *fibula* may damage the peroneal nerve, and this diagnosis is easy. In contrast, pressure injury of the nerve by a plaster cast is often overlooked if the doctor does not pay attention to complaints of paresthesia or pain on the dorsal aspect of the foot directly behind the first and second toes, or to weakness in the elevation (extension) of the big (first) toe.

16.1.4 Iatrogenic Paralysis Owing to Incorrect Intramuscular Injection. Another instance of *iatrogenic damage* is incorrect intramuscular injection into the buttocks. The division of the sciatic nerve into its main branches, the peroneal and tibial nerves, is sometimes quite proximal, so that only the peroneal nerve is affected. Roughly 10% of patients do not experience the ominous paresthesia and pain during or immediately after the injection, and the onset of weakness may be delayed. These are complicated legal cases, and the doctor will maintain that the footdrop was caused by the condition under treatment, i.e., lumbar radiculopathy. There is a simple way of distinguishing between a lesion at the level of the lumbar roots and in the peripheral course of the sciatic nerve. The lumbar roots do not carry sympathetic fibers for the innervation of sweat glands. These leave the spinal cord no more caudally than at the level of L-2, and join the sciatic nerve only at an intrapelvic location, from which they travel to the periphery. Absence of sweating in the distribution area of the sciatic nerve or its branches clearly indicates a peripheral lesion.

16.1.5 Herniated Lumbar Disc. Unilateral footdrop may be due to herniation of a lumbar disc. The event is not always abrupt and painful, and tenderness of the back or a positive Lasègue's sign are not essential. If only the fifth lumbar root is affected, the ankle jerk may be present, although all the above-mentioned findings, or rather absence of findings, are present. The muscle supply of the fifth root, however, is not identical with that of the peroneal nerve. So the distinction can be made on the basis of careful examination and some knowledge of anatomy.

16.1.6 Diabetic and Alcoholic Neuropathy. Finally, it should be mentioned that there are instances of *polyneuropathy* where the patient presents with unilateral footdrop, whereas affection of other nerves is subclinical, or almost so. This is seen in diabetes mellitus and in chronic alcohol abuse. As a rule, however, there is at least a bilateral diminution of ankle jerks.

16.1.7 Syndrome of the Anterior Tibial Artery. The term syndrome of the anterior tibial artery denotes ischemic damage of the long extensor muscles of the foot and toes (anterior tibial and extensor digitorum communis muscles). These lie in a narrow compartment formed dorsally by the anterior aspect of the tibia and ventrally by a tight fascia. Embolic or thrombotic occlusion of the anterior tibial artery results in edematous swelling of the muscles. As the fascia cannot give way, the swelling leads to compression of the capillaries and, finally, to ischemic necrosis of the muscles, together with ischemic damage to the anterior tibial nerve. A similar mechanism may be triggered by abnormal strain on the muscles, e.g., during a game of soccer or a long walk.

Signs and symptoms are painful swelling of the pretibial region, followed by weakness of extension that becomes complete within a few hours. The dorsal artery of the foot is, as a rule, pulseless. Diagnosis must be made before onset of muscular paralysis, because the only effective therapy is generous surgical incision of the fascia in order to relieve the compression.

16.2 Central

A rather circumscribed cortical or subcortical lesion is indicated by central footdrop.

16.2.1 Ischemic Infarction and Brain Tumor. Acute onset is suggestive of ischemic infarction, whereas chronic evolution is characteristic of brain tumor. The level of blood pressure may be misleading because, of course, hypertensive persons also develop primary or metastatic brain tumor. On the other hand, headache and mental alteration may occur only at a rather late stage in the growth of a cerebral malignancy. So one should always contemplate both alternatives and subject the patient to neuroimaging examination, if possible. Considering the therapeutic consequences, this measure appears fully justified.

16.2.2 Postparoxysmal Paresis. Any kind of transient weakness may be a postparoxysmal phenomenon, where the (partial or generalized) seizure has gone unrecognized. Serum creatine kinase is often but not always elevated in these cases. Focal signs during or following a seizure should prompt a thorough search for a space-occupying or vascular brain lesion.

17 Horner's Syndrome

Horner's syndrome is due to damage to the sympathetic pathway anywhere in its long course from the diencephalon down to the lateral gray in the upper thoracic spinal cord, and up again through the neck to the eye and upper eyelid. This pathway has three neurons. The central neuron passes from the hypothalamus through the posterolateral brain stem to the lateral gray in the spinal cord (Clarke's column), ending at the level T1. The peripheral *presynaptic* neuron travels up the cervical sympathetic chain to end in its superior cervical ganglion. The peripheral *postsynaptic* neuron runs up on the surface of the carotid artery and branches off toward the eye at the level of the orbit to innervate the pupil, the upper eyelid, and the blood vessels of the eye, in particular those of the conjunctiva.

Horner's syndrome has the following features:

- Miosis of medium degree in the presence of normal pupillary reactions to light and accommodation/near sight
- Slight ptosis which, in contrast to third nerve palsy, is never complete
- Dilation of the conjunctival vessels

Frequently, there is sudomotor disturbance of varying extension (see below). Enophthalmus is not present, although older textbooks state the contrary.

The diagnosis of the disease process causing Horner's syndrome is largely dependent on the localization of the lesion in the sympathetic pathway. Localization is accomplished by considering both the neurologic symptoms that may accompany Horner's syndrome and the results of some simple pharmacologic tests which may demonstrate denervation hypersensitivity of the pupil, which is indicative of damage to the third sympathetic neuron. These tests have a value only when localization is not suggested by neurologic signs, i.e., in those rare cases where Horner's syndrome appears in isolation.

17.1 Central Horner's Syndrome in Brain Stem and Medullary Lesions

There is ipsilateral Horner's syndrome plus ipsilateral diminution of sweating on the whole of one side of the body. Owing to the neighborhood of the efferent, uncrossed sympathetic and the afferent, crossed spinothalamic pathways, there is frequently impairment in sensation of pain and temperature on the contralateral half of the body. The level of damage in the brain stem can be recognized by gaze or cranial nerve paralysis and impairment of the pathways connecting the brain stem and the cerebellum. Paralysis of horizontal gaze indicates a pontine lesion, as do fifth, sixth, and seventh nerve palsy. The caudal group of cranial nerves is affected in medullary lesions. Textbooks tend to describe characteristic "crossed brain stem syndromes" bearing venerable names and allegedly of great localizing value. This is not our experience, and it also does not fit modern views on the pathophysiology of vascular brain stem disease.

17.1.1 Ischemic Stroke. By far the largest diagnostic group is ischemic stroke. This is due to embolic infarction, or atherosclerosis of large vessels supplying the brain stem, or autochthonous occlusion owing to small-vessel disease of mostly hypertensive origin. It cannot reasonably be expected that this kind of disease will produce only one focal brain stem lesion. Furthermore, the great variability of brain stem vascularization makes the occurrence of prototypical syndromes most unlikely. Even Wallenberg's lateral medullary syndrome is observed more often than not in "atypical" variations of the original description. The basic combination of signs that points to the brain stem is: ipsilateral cranial nerve dysfunction, ipsilateral Horner's syndrome, if present, ipsi- or contralateral cerebellar ataxia, and contralateral hemiparesis and/or sensory loss.

17.1.2 Multiple Sclerosis. Similar considerations hold true for multiple sclerosis, which, however, rarely gives rise to a central Horner's syndrome. The diagnosis of multiple sclerosis is discussed in Chap. 10.

17.1.3 Primary or Metastatic Brain Stem Tumors. Primary or metastatic brain stem tumors are mostly located in the midbrain or pons, and may cause Horner's syndrome. The diagnosis is made by considering the progressive evolution of signs and symptoms that can be attributed to one relatively circumscribed area of the brain stem. Neuroimaging and electrophysiological studies are needed in the first place to confirm the diagnosis.

17.1.4 Cavity of Syringomyelia or Intramedullary Tumor. In the lower brain stem and upper spinal cord Horner's syndrome may be caused by a cavity of syringomyelia or an intramedullary tumor of the same location, i.e., centrally placed in the medulla oblongata or the spinal cord. The outstanding features are Horner's syndrome, ipsilateral disturbance of thermoregulatory sweating, and contralateral loss of sensation of pain and temperature. If the anterior horn of the spinal cord is affected, there may be ipsilateral progressive wasting of hand muscles (see Chap. 27). Central paraparesis may also be present, but bladder dysfunction is rare.

17.2 Peripheral Horner's Syndrome

17.2.1 Preganglionic (Mostly Thoracic or Neck Malignancy). After leaving the spinal cord via the first thoracic root, the sympathetic fibers join the cervical sympathetic chain. At the proximal end this pathway may be damaged by apical carcinoma of the lung (Pancoast's tumor). Only when detected early is this tumor susceptible to combined radiological and surgical treatment. A very characteristic combination is throbbing pain in the axilla, and later on down the arm, and ipsilateral Horner's syndrome. Sweating is impaired in the ipsilateral face and shoulder region. As the tumor expands, it eventually invades the brachial plexus. Pain at this stage becomes worse, and wasting of the small hand muscles develops.

Other causes, e.g., a cervical rib, are extremely rare.

Higher up, at the neck, the sympathetic chain may be damaged by metastatic infiltration of lymph nodes, by surgical extirpation of these, or, rarely, by thyroid carcinoma. In these cases there is Horner's syndrome without denervation hypersensitivity to epinephrine (see below), ipsilateral impairment of sweating in the area indicated above for Pancoast's tumor, but no signs of affection of the brachial plexus. Local pain is mild or absent. The preganglionic site of lesion is demonstrated by the effect of cocaine in a 2% solution. The dilating action of cocaine on the pupil depends on the integrity of the third sympathetic neuron and, consequently, on the presence of amine oxidase at the endings of the sympathetic fibers in the iris. Only in preganglionic Horner's syndrome will there be the mydriasis which is expected following instillation of cocaine at the conjunctiva.

17.2.2 Postganglionic (Processes at the Base of the Skull and in the Orbit). This is not accompanied by sudomotor disturbance. Local application of cocaine to the eye has no effect. There is denervation hypersensitivity with decrease of amine oxidase. Application of epinephrine in a 0.1% solution is followed with a latency of roughly 20 min by medium-sized mydriasis, whereas this low concentration of epinephrine has no effect on the normal eye.

There are various disease processes to be considered, which have in common their localization close to the internal carotid artery where it traverses the base of the skull and the cavernous sinus, and close to the third nerve and the nasociliary branch of the fifth nerve as they travel to the eye. Most important are parasellar granulomatous or neoplastic processes, and tumor or inflammatory disease of the orbit. Once the clinical localization has been established, only ancillary examinations will reveal the diagnosis. The most promising tool is neuroimaging with contrast.

18 "Hypersomnia"

Hypersomnia occurs in two ways: some patients fall asleep frequently and in inappropriate situations, while others sleep all the time when left alone. Their condition is distinct from coma, however, in that they can be aroused relatively easily.

18.1 Narcoleptic Attacks

A characteristic feature of narcoleptic attacks is an irresistible urge to sleep that befalls the patient several times a day. Occurrence of the attacks is not limited to resting situations, such as sitting in a chair and reading or watching television. Even while the patient is moving about and/or doing some work that normally attracts his attention, he may suddenly feel the imperative need to sit down and have a nap. Many patients are able to marshall all their strength in order to postpone the attack somewhat, but they will not succeed in avoiding it. Some persons develop strategies to keep the attacks secret, e.g., going to the toilet. These strategies are facilitated by the fact that the attack of sleep usually lasts no more than a few minutes, after which the patient wakes up and feels reposed. In rare instances, instead of falling asleep the patient exhibits automatic behavior, with continuation of complex actions he was engaged in at the onset of the narcoleptic attack.

Some patients have only narcoleptic attacks. Others also have cataplectic attacks, which involve a sudden and very brief loss of muscular tone. If only the arms are affected, the patient may drop an object he is holding or handling. If there is generalized loss of tone he may abruptly kneel down, or nearly so. The cataplectic attacks are provoked by any sudden emotional reaction, such as laughing at a joke or being startled.

A third phenomenon experienced by some narcoleptic patients is called "sleep paralysis." While lying in bed and about to fall asleep, the patient is suddenly unable to move his limbs or to utter a sound, although his mind is wide awake. This is described as a most alarming event because the patient is afraid his respiration might cease (which it does not), yet he has no means of communicating. The attack abates by itself or if by chance the patient is touched or spoken to. Similar attacks may occur during the night or in the morning. Most patients have an unsound sleep, and they remember violent dreams.

The diagnosis of narcolepsy is arrived at mainly by careful history taking. Neurologic and medical findings are unremarkable. EEG is most helpful. Most, if not all, narcoleptic patients fall asleep as soon as the recording starts, and usually reach stage C without much delay. Patients with cataplexy have so-called sleep-onset REM periods early in the recording (REM, rapid eye movement). All-night EEG recording shows a quite irregular pattern, similar to that of infants and suggestive of lack of maturation of the sleep mechanisms.

18.2 Pickwickian Syndrome (Sleep Apnea Syndrome)

The best-known variant of the so-called sleep apnea syndrome, pickwickian syndrome, is easily distinguished from narcolepsy. The patients fall asleep only when they are sitting and have nothing particular to do. While they are sleeping, breathing excursions become flatter and slower, and finally stop. After an apneic period of variable length they resume breathing with a loud snore. The apneic periods also occur during sleep, and the recurrent loud snores may be heard even in another room. The patients are quite obese, often hypertensive, and there is hypercapnia and compensatory polyglobulia.

18.3 Intoxication

Continuous somnolence is quite suggestive of a state of intoxication. The suspicion is corroborated when the patient also has slurred speech. Nystagmus is a frequent but not mandatory sign, as is ataxia. Beta activity in the EEG usually supports the diagnosis earlier than toxicologic examination of blood and urine specimens.

18.4 Metabolic Derangement

Almost any kind of metabolic derangement may render the patient somnolent. The medical diagnoses cannot be discussed here in detail. One frequent cause, dehydration in elderly persons, should, however, be stressed. This is a very common finding when the neurologic consultant is called to a patient who has been operated on and is deteriorating for no obvious reason. Elevation of hematocrit is quite frequently found in these cases.

18.5 Organic Disease of the Upper Brain Stem and Diencephalon

Every organic brain disease that is located in the upper brain stem may leave the patient somnolent. There are primary and metastatic tumors, occlusion of the basilar artery or of some of its branches, bilateral thalamic infarctions, and hypertensive hemorrhage of the brain stem. If neurologic findings point to the locus of lesion, neuroimaging examination is required. When there is neither hemorrhage nor direct or indirect (occlusive hydrocephalus) evidence of tumor, EEG and evoked potential studies should be performed, while at the same time the neuroradiologist prepares for angiography. It is our experience that after careful consideration every available ancillary examination should be applied in the case of these patients.

One condition, however, can frequently be diagnosed on clinical grounds alone. This is the case of the patient who after a long period of alcohol abuse becomes drowsy and exhibits ocular signs, such as unequal pupils, partial or complete third nerve palsy, nystagmus, and ataxia. This syndrome permits the diagnosis of Wernicke's encephalopathy (see Chap. 6). Neuroimaging is useful, because the patient may, in addition, have bilateral pachymengingeosis. If neuroimaging shows only the usual reduction in cerebral and cerebellar volume, high-dosage intravenous or intramuscular vitamin B_1 treatment should be given prior to invasive diagnostic measures.

18.6 Kleine-Levin Syndrome

A rare condition is the hypersomnia in adolescent males called Kleine-Levin syndrome. Periods of uninterrupted sleep for several days and nights alternate with short bouts of wakefulness during which the patients exhibit bulimia, i.e., they consume great quantities of food. On neurologic examination there are no abnormal findings, and EEG is normal during the waking state. The condition eventually resolves, and is assumed to be of psychic origin.

18.7 Psychogenic Somnolence

Somnolence of psychogenic origin also occurs without periods of bulimia. Usually, the patients do not appear to be completely asleep. If they do, EEG shows clearly that they are, in fact, awake. On neurologic examination they will avert their eyes if one tries to lift their eyelids. The muscle tone is usually flaccid, and there may be no reaction to mildly painful or startling stimuli that would normally arouse a patient with somnolence of organic origin. Psychogenic somnolence resolves after at most several days.

19 Impairment in Anteflexion of the Head

Impairment in the anteflexion of the head has three possible causes. The most common is reflex contraction of the muscles of the neck, owing to a disease of the meninges called cervical rigidity. The meninges have a very rich innervation by sensory nerves, and any traction of the meninges by anteflexion of the head may cause severe pain. Consequently, reflex contraction of the neck muscles counteracts anteflexion, and sometimes maintains the head in a retracted position. A similar mechanism is at work in space-occupying lesions of the posterior fossa. Muscular rigidity may be strong enough to prevent not only active, but also passive head movements.

Finally, there is a variety of osseous diseases that lead to a fixation of the upper vertebral column.

19.1 Meningitis

19.1.1 Acute Purulent. It is relatively easily to recognize acute purulent meningitis if the patient is bedridden and febrile, complains of severe headache, and has photophobia. Cervical rigidity is present in an early stage, and head retraction and a tendency to lie in a general flexor position are observed as the process of infection of the meninges progresses. Usually Kernig's and Brudzinski's signs can be elicited, both of which involve movements that cause traction of the nerve roots embedded in the inflammatory exudate. In acute purulent meningitis the patient usually appears obtuse, is frequently delirious, and may become comatose. These general signs and symptoms may be accompanied by reflex changes, plantar extensor responses, cranial nerve palsy, and jacksonian fits, which will not be discussed here in detail.

CSF contains many thousands of polymorphonuclear cells, a high level of protein, and a low level of glucose, with a corresponding increase in lactate. Microorganisms are demonstrated microscopically or by culture.

19.1.2 Chronic. In contrast, chronic meningitis, e.g., that caused by *Mycobacterium tuberculosis* or by fungi, is quite hard to diagnose, because frequently all of the above-mentioned signs and symptoms are quite attenuated. It is beyond the scope of this book to give a differential diagnosis of the various types of meningitis which are due to microorganisms.

19.1.3 Lymphocytic and Aseptic. The terms lymphocytic meningitis and aseptic meningitis are interchangeably applied to meningitis, or rather to meningoencephalitis of viral origin. Onset is acute in most cases, and the initial signs and symptoms resemble those of purulent meningitis, with the exception that there is a somewhat lower level of fever and lesser frequency of delirium. Coma is not observed, and neurologic signs other than cranial nerve palsy are very rarely seen.

CSF shows pleocytosis mainly of mononuclear cells, with a smaller proportion of polymorphonuclear cells during the first few days. Elevation of the protein level is not excessive, glucose content is normal, and the lactate level is fairly low.

19.1.4 Carcinomatous and Leukemic. Cervical rigidity in an afebrile patient who shows signs of general illness should arouse suspicion of carcinomatous meningitis, especially if a severe, throbbing, and spontaneous headache is present. It is not a prerequisite that systemic cancer be known or found on routine examination. Even standard laboratory findings may be in the normal range.

This is not true for leukemic meningitis, where laboratory findings are quite often suggestive of hematological disease, even if they reveal only an abnormally low level of thrombocytic cells, or disturbance in hemostaseological mechanisms. The CSF often contains tumor cells. The protein level, as a rule, is elevated, the glucose level reduced, and the lactate level correspondingly high.

19.2 Subarachnoid Hemorrhage (SAH)

The clinical picture of SAH is described in Chap. 4. Onset is acute, the leading symptom is headache of a severity that the patient has never experienced before, and there is cervical rigidity. Kernig's and Brudzinski's signs are not always positive in the initial stage. Lumbar tap reveals sanguinolent CSF. The supernatant fluid is colored yellow, provided the event took place more than five hours previously. For further diagnostic procedures and findings, see Chap. 4.

19.3 Tumors of the Posterior Fossa or of the Craniospinal Junction

Forced flexion of the head and sometimes also lateral tilt are seen in posterior fossa and craniospinal junction tumors, and there is also reflex resistance to passive movements of the head. There is no fever or photophobia. As a rule the patients have a long history of headache, frequently treated by chiropractic procedures. At the stage discussed here they are prone to vomit spontaneously and upon movements of the head. Papilledema is frequent, except in hemangioblastoma. Some patients have paresthesias in both hands, owing to dorsal column irritation. Neuroimaging techniques establish the diagnosis.

19.4 Parkinson's Disease

Muscular rigidity in Parkinson's disease is found particularly in the neck. As a result, anteflexion and passive rotation of the head have to overcome muscular resistance that is often painful, because as time goes on the forced "stoop" leads to stiffness in the intervertebral joints, which are richly supplied with sensory nerves. The American neurologist, Robert Wartenberg, has proposed to use this stiffness of the neck for the early diagnosis of parkinsonism. If the doctor places the patient flat on the bed or the examination couch, lifts the head passively some 30°, and suddenly withdraws his support, the parkinsonian patient's head will not fall back abruptly, but rather sink back to the horizontal very slowly.

19.5 Progressive Supranuclear Palsy

Neck rigidity is a prominent symptom in progressive supranuclear palsy, a rare degenerative disease of unknown etiology. The leading symptoms are paralysis of downward gaze, developing slowly to complete gaze paralysis in all directions, accompanied or followed by parkinsonian rigidity and akinesia.

19.6 Vertebral Disease at the Cervical Level
Including Bechterew's Disease (Ankylosing Spondylitis)

Any vertebral disease of the cervical spine will, of course, impair active and passive movements. Attempts to overcome the resistance are painful, but there is little spontaneous pain. The patients are afebrile and do not appear generally ill. The most important disease to affect the vertebrae is ankylosing spondylitis, diagnosis of which is made by radiological examination and demonstration of HLA-B27.

20 Lesions of Cranial Nerves, Bilateral

The conditions discussed in this chapter have an acute or subacute evolution. Pain may be prominent or absent, which provides an important diagnostic clue. The disease processes affect either the meninges or the brain stem, or both. CSF examination is therefore mandatory, and should include cell count, determination of the type of cells, assessment of the levels of protein, glucose, lactate, and immunoglobulins, and the search for bacteria or other microorganisms.

20.1 Carcinomatous or Leukemic Meningitis

The onset of carcinomatous or leukemic meningitis is insidious. Many patients complain of severe headache that is not alleviated by conventional analgesic drugs. Neck stiffness is often mild or absent, and sometimes the primary malignancy has not yet been recognized. Diagnosis rests on CSF examination. Typical findings are: mild pleocytosis consisting of "atypical" or tumor cells, a disproportionate elevation of the protein level, and a reduced glucose level with subsequent elevation of the lactate level. Almost identical protein, glucose, and lactate findings are seen in sarcoidosis and tuberculous meningitis. The demonstration of tumor cells or the detection of a malignancy, e.g., of breast or lung cancer, is therefore of the utmost importance.

20.2 Tuberculous Meningitis

The incidence of tuberculous meningitis has increased during the last few years. Its onset is even more insidious than that of carcinomatous meningitis, headache being mild, if present at all. The same holds true for neck stiffness. Quite frequently, patients give the overall impression of being ill. Pulmonary X-ray may be unremarkable. CSF shows mild lymphocytic pleocytosis and increased protein, grossly reduced glucose, and elevation of lactate. If microscopic examination reveals the presence of mycobacteria, the diagnosis is easy. More frequently, however, one has to wait for confirmation by animal inoculation tests. It is essential that tuberculostatic therapy is not postponed until these findings are available, but is initiated as soon as the diagnosis is suspected.

20.3 Sarcoidosis

The diagnosis of sarcoidosis is extremely difficult. The clinical picture is quite similar to tuberculous meningitis, as are the CSF findings. An important finding is a negative cutaneous Tine test, indicating lack of reactivity to *Mycobacterium tuberculosis*. Radiological investigation of the lungs, hands, or feet may reveal systemic affection by the disease. If there is swelling of lymphatic nodules or enlargement of the mediastinum, histological examination may provide the diagnosis.

20.4 Syphilitic Affection of the CNS

A diagnosis which still – or again – should be considered is syphilitic affection of the CNS, especially when there is bilateral paralysis of ocular movements. Frequently, the pupils are unequal in width, and an important sign is the absence of pupillary reaction to light. Reaction to near sight/convergence may or may not be preserved. Blood tests for the activity of syphilitic disease are strongly positive, and CSF shows elevation of the levels of lymphocytic cells and protein, and autochthonous production of IgG (see Chap. 10).

20.5 Lyme Disease

A triad of bilateral facial palsy, asymmetrical polyneuropathy, and chronic meningitis is called Lyme disease. Some patients have in addition painful arthritis and myocarditis. Many patients report that the neurologic symptoms were preceded by a dermatological affection, erythema chronicum migrans, originating from the part of the body where they have been bitten by a tick. CSF contains raised cell and protein levels.

It has recently been recognized that the disease is caused by a tick-transmitted spirochete, which can be identified by specific IgG and IgM antibodies in serum and CSF. An immunofluorescent test is also available. The infection responds favorably to penicillin.

20.6 Brain Stem Encephalitis (Bickerstaff's Encephalitis)

The onset of brain stem encephalitis is usually marked by decreased vigilance. This is followed by bilateral affection of the cranial nerves in a descending course. There is usually paralysis of the oculomotor, trigeminal, facial, accessory, and hypoglossal nerves. In addition, there are frank brain stem signs, such as gaze paralysis, ataxia, and plantar extensor signs. The evolution is very dramatic, especially when the patient becomes somnolent. Yet rarely, if ever, is there respiratory failure, and the prognosis is good provided there are no pulmonary or thrombotic complications. CSF findings are similar to those in Guillain-Barré or Miller Fisher's syndrome.

20.7 Guillain-Barré Syndrome

Only brief mention need be made here of Guillain-Barré syndrome. Usually, bilateral paralysis of the facial, trigeminal, accessory, or hypoglossal nerves occurs after the development of flaccid paraparesis with – often delayed – areflexia and slowing of nerve conduction (see also Chap. 34). CSF shows a normal cell count with elevation of the protein level. In these cases, the diagnosis has been established before the onset of cranial nerve paralysis. Only very rarely does paralysis of cranial nerves herald the disease: in these cases repeated measurement of nerve conduction velocity is of great diagnostic help, because the disease affects primarily the myelin sheaths.

20.8 Miller Fisher's Syndrome

The course of events is different in Miller Fisher's syndrome, which is considered a variant of Guillain-Barré syndrome, or at least quite closely related to it. The patients develop an *external* ophthalmoplegia, which eventually becomes complete. Limb movements become ataxic, and proprioceptive reflexes are lost. Flaccid paralyses are not usually severe. In some cases, however, a frank Guillain-Barré polyneuritis is combined with tetraplegia, and possibly respiratory failure and autonomic neuropathy (see Chap. 34) with external ophthalmoplegia.

20.9 Wernicke's Encephalopathy

In contrast, Wernicke's encephalopathy affects the autonomic and the somatic innervation of the eyes. The patients have dilated pupils that hardly react to light, and various oculomotor signs ranging from incomplete paralysis of the third nerve with diplopia to horizontal or vertical gaze paralysis. There is cerebellar ataxia, and reactivity may be decreased (see also Chaps. 6 and 10). Since most cases of Wernicke's encephalopathy are due to chronic alcohol abuse with depletion of vitamin B_1, the patients are likely to exhibit signs of polyneuropathy.

The distinction from Miller Fisher's syndrome, which is important for therapy, rests on the following signs: autonomic third nerve paralysis is suggestive of Wernicke's disease, and in polyneuropathy which is due to alcohol abuse there is only a moderate decrease in nerve conduction velocity, while in Miller Fisher's syndrome, as in Guillain-Barré syndrome, nerve conduction is slow and there are no gross signs of muscular denervation.

21 Lesions of Cranial Nerves, Unilateral

Unilateral paralyses of cranial nerves that have a close topographical relationship are indicative of neoplastic or inflammatory disease of the base of the skull. As will be seen, their localizing value is of great help in detecting the underlying disease processes.

21.1 Anterior Fossa Syndrome

A disease process in the anterior fossa will affect the olfactory and the optic nerve. In contrast to bilateral anosmia, which grossly interferes with the synesthetic perception of the flavor of food and beverages, unilateral anosmia is not usually spontaneously noticed by the patient. The same holds true, in many cases, for monocular impairment of vision. As a rule, it is the alteration in the patient's personality that prompts the family to seek the doctor's advice. He will find the patient lacking in spontaneity, emotionally flat, and sometimes unduly jocular. At that stage there is pallor of the optic disc, and monocular vision is close to zero. Illumination of the affected eye fails to produce consensual constriction of the opposite pupil, while the affected eye shows normal pupillary constriction when the healthy eye is illuminated. There is ipsilateral loss of the sense of smell.

In most instances the syndrome is caused by a brain tumor which is usually a meningioma at the bottom of the anterior fossa.

21.2 Sphenoid Wing Syndrome

Tumors of the sphenoid wing, mostly meningiomas, lead to a very characteristic combination of signs and symptoms. The patient complains of continuous unilateral headache in the temporal bone or in the orbit. There may be nonpulsating exophthalmus, which can be recognized by comparing the positions of two spatulae placed horizontally on the patient's closed eyes. There is paralysis of the nerves that travel through the sphenoid fissure, i.e., the oculomotor, trochlear, and abducent nerves, and sensory disturbance in the ophthalmic branch of the trigeminal nerve. Consequently, the patient has diplopia in various directions, and movements of the globe are grossly impaired. The corneal reflex is absent, and there is hypesthesia on the ipsilateral front and bridge of the nose.

21.3 Foster Kennedy Syndrome

Although well known to many medical students, Foster Kennedy syndrome is very rarely encountered in medical practice. Allegedly, there is ipsilateral atrophy of the optic nerve with pallor of the optic disc, while on the contralateral side there is papilledema. The syndrome is said to be caused by a meningioma growing on the medial side of the sphenoid wing.

21.4 Apex of the Orbit Syndrome

The apex of the orbit syndrome has practical importance. There is primary atrophy of the optic nerve with sharply demarcated pallor of the optic disc. In addition, all those nerves that pass through the sphenoid fissure are paralyzed, as explained in Sect. 21.2. The maxillary branch of the trigeminal nerve leaves the base of the skull through the foramen rotundum, the mandibular branch through the foramen ovale.

This syndrome is seen in inflammatory and in neoplastic (primary or metastatic) disease.

21.5 Syndrome of the Cavernous Sinus

In the cavernous sinus syndrome, again, all three nerves acting on the ocular muscles are affected to varying degrees. There is also hypesthesia in the first branch of the trigeminal nerve, but no affection of the optic nerve. The eye may show signs of congestion due to impairment of the venous outflow from the orbit to the cavernous sinus.

Etiology is manifold: infraclinoid meningioma, infraclinoid aneurysm of the internal carotid artery, thrombosis of the cavernous sinus, and spontaneous or traumatic fistula between the carotid artery and the cavernous sinus. The syndrome is also seen in Tolosa-Hunt syndrome, a granulomatous inflammatory disease that responds favorably to corticosteroid therapy (see Chap. 6).

21.6 Gradenigo's Syndrome (Lesion at the Apex of the Petrous Bone)

Although of good localizing value, Gradenigo's syndrome is rare. Inflammatory disease of the petrous bone may affect the trigeminal, abducent, and facial nerves.

21.7 Syndrome of the Cerebellopontine Angle

One cannot adequately describe the syndrome of the cerebellopontine angle in a static way, i.e., without considering its very characteristic evolution, which is invariably due to tumor (acoustic neuroma, meningioma, epidermoid cyst). Usually, the first symptom is impairment in the auditory perception of higher frequencies, which is noticed when the telephone is used. Next, tinnitus develops. Vertigo is infrequent, but if it is present it is an unsystematic dizziness, and definitely not of the paroxysmal rotatory Menière type.

Nystagmus is very common. In the initial stage it is directed toward the healthy ear, as is characteristic for a chronic peripheral labyrinthine lesion, which can be demonstrated by caloric tests. In an advanced stage of the disease, pressure on the pontine reticular formation of the brainstem leads to central nystagmus that beats in the direction of (ipsilateral or contralateral) sideward gaze.

Next, the opthalmic and maxillary branches of the trigeminal nerve are affected, with ipsilateral loss of the corneal reflex and pain and/or hypesthesia on the cheek. The facial nerve is regularly paralyzed. Sometimes, irritation of the nerve leads to paroxysmal hemifacial spasm (see Chap. 13). Paralysis of the abducent nerve gives rise to diplopia that increases when the gaze is directed toward the side of the lesion. Increasing pressure on the pons results in ipsilateral locomotor hemiataxia. At that stage, the patient complains of severe headache, and he may have vestibular tilt of the head toward the side of the lesion (see Chap. 10).

21.8 Syndrome of the Jugular Foramen

Any disease process in the region of the foramen jugulare interferes with the functions of the glossopharyngeal, vagal and hypoglossal nerves. The glossopharyngeal is for all practical purposes a purely sensory nerve. The patients either have hypesthesia in the palatal and/or pharyngeal region, or experience attacks of glossopharyngeal neuralgia. This rare neuralgia consists in paroxysmal pain in the region of the tonsils or in the middle ear, which extends toward the pharynx. The attacks may be accompanied by coughing, and are triggered by swallowing, speaking, and drinking cold beverages. Paralysis of the tenth (vagal) nerve is usually complete, i.e., there is not only hoarseness of the voice due to affection of the recurrent branch of the nerve, but also paralysis of the soft palate, which interferes with the production of sounds that require closure of the nasal cavity, such as "m" or "n".

Beverages may be regurgitated through the nose; unilateral hypoglossal paralysis slightly impedes swallowing; and speech becomes somewhat awkward. The outstretched tongue is pushed toward the side of the lesion by the nonparalyzed muscle, while in the resting position deviation toward the affected side may be observed, as well as hemiatrophy with fibrillations. The syndrome is caused by metastatic tumors or by the rare glomus jugulare tumor.

21.9 Syndrome of the Cervico-Occipital Junction

Metastatic tumors or malformations of the cervico-occipital junction lead to a combination of cranial nerve lesions and symptoms owing to affection of the cervical portion of the spinal cord. The cranial nerves involved are the glossopharyngeal, vagus, accessory (ipsilateral paralysis of sternomastoid and upper portion of trapezius muscles), and hypoglossal nerves. In addition, there are signs and symptoms indicating involvement of the pyramidal tract and the dorsal columns, mainly numbness and paresthesia in the distal portions of the lower and upper extremities, and central paresis of the hands and legs.

21.10 Garcin's Syndrome

Malignant tumors of the epipharynx invade the base of the skull from outside. Upon penetrating the cranial cavity they produce unilateral lesions of neighboring cranial nerves that do not conform the syndromes described above. This combination was first pointed out by the French neurologist, Garcin. There may be involvement of the trigeminal (sensory, as well as motor), facial, statoacoustic, glossopharyngeal, accessory, and hypoglossal nerves.

The clinical picture is quite characteristic. Neuroimaging of the base of the skull confirms the diagnosis. Inspection of the epipharynx may reveal the presence of a local malignancy. Biopsy and/or examination of CSF may yield positive cytologic findings that reveal the nature of the malignancy.

22 Monocular Loss of Vision

Whether the loss of vision in one eye has an abrupt onset or a slowly progressive evolution, the patient will probably first seek advice from an ophthalmologist. Yet, as in acute blindness, i.e., bilateral loss of vision, the underlying cause in the majority of cases is neurologic in nature.

22.1 Acute Conditions

22.1.1 Amaurosis Fugax. In the elderly, the most frequent condition of sudden and transient monocular loss of vision is appropriately termed amaurosis fugax. Unilateral blindness or severely blurred vision befalls the patient without warning and usually lasts for several minutes or as much as half a day. Routine ophthalmologic examination is usually conducted only after the condition has cleared and will most probably reveal nothing remarkable except some degree of arteriosclerosis of the retinal vessels, which is not unusual in persons of this age. As a rule, the patient's reading glasses are corrected, and he is reassured that nothing serious has happened to his eyes.

In more than 90% of cases, amaurosis fugax is due to an embolus originating from an ulcerating plaque of the ipsilateral internal carotid artery at the neck and carried by the bloodstream into the ophthalmic artery. The ensuing ischemia leads to a breakdown of visual function. Usually the embolus is carried further into a peripheral retinal arterial branch, while at the same time spontaneous thrombolysis takes place; hence the rapid resolution of symptoms.

During the acute stage, this course of events can be recognized by a collapsed retinal artery, or because fluorescent angiography permits direct visualization of the embolus as it travels toward the periphery of the retina. Rarely, however, will this examination be available.

Since an attack of amaurosis fugax is followed by a completed hemispheric stroke in 30% of cases before a year has elapsed, it is of vital importance for the patient that the doctor is familiar with the condition. Doppler ultrasound sonography (A-scan or B-scan) is the examination of choice in these cases and the ulcerated stenosis of the carotid should be operated on without delay.

22.1.2 Ophthalmic Migraine. In young persons, an attack of ophthalmic migraine may lead to a similar condition, and, as explained in Chap. 4, the headache may be minor and escape attention, especially since amaurosis is such an alarming event. Doppler ultrasonography is useful also in these cases, because in migraine it will be normal. On the other hand, there is one arterial disease, so-called fibromuscular dysplasia, which may cause neurologic symptoms and signs well ahead of the age at which incipient stroke is expected.

22.2 Subacute or Chronic Progressive Conditions

22.2.1 Optic Neuritis and Retrobulbar Neuritis. Subacute monocular deterioration of vision in younger individuals without headache and with normal ultrasound findings is strongly suggestive of neuritis of the optic nerve. Depending on the extent to which the nerve is affected, the patient will be virtually blind in one eye, which is very rare, or will report seeing the visual world as though through an opaque medium, or not being able to read fine print, a frequent phenomenon which is due to affection of the maculopapillary bundle deep in the course of the optic nerve.

If the optic disc is swollen, brain tumor may be suspected. Papilledema, however, leaves vision intact for a long period of time, in marked contrast to optic neuritis, where loss of vision is present right at the beginning. In retrobulbar neuritis, the inflammatory process takes place in the retro-orbital part of the nerve, as the term implies. Consequently, ophthalmoscopic findings are normal in the acute stage; hence the saying that neither the patient nor the doctor can see anything. Recording of visually evoked potentials (VEPs) will demonstrate functional disturbance in the optic nerve. Optic or retrobulbar neuritis is in roughly 30% of cases the first manifestation of multiple sclerosis, and it may also occur in the later course of the disease. If it is known that the patient has multiple sclerosis there will be no diagnostic problems. If not, one should carefully inquire for typical symptoms of the disease and examine the overall neurologic status (see Chap. 10). Also, in this case the full program of electrophysiological examinations is called for: bilateral examination of VEPs, the blink reflex, and somatosensory evoked potentials (SSEPs) following stimulation of the median and the tibial nerves with a view to testing the functioning of those pathways most frequently affected by the disease.

If optic neuritis appears in the initial stage of multiple sclerosis, then unfortunately the search for multiple localization of dysfunction will yield normal results. For reasons discussed in Chap. 6, I do not recommend routine examination of CSF under these circumstances. The younger the patient, the greater the likelihood of evolving multiple slcerosis.

22.2.2 Ischemic Retinopathy. In old age, ischemic damage to the optic nerve and retina may cause similar signs and symptoms. Demonstration of impaired arterial perfusion requires fluorescent angiography. Frequently, there is atherosclerotic narrowing of the internal carotid artery.

22.2.3 "Alcohol-Tobacco" Amblyopia (i.e., Vitamin B_{12} Deficiency). The so-called alcohol-tobacco amblyopia may begin with deterioration of vision in one eye, although eventually both eyes will be affected, The term is somewhat misleading. The cause of the disease is neither the toxic effect of tobacco nor of alcohol, but rather a lack of vitamin B_{12}. Deficient availability of the vitamin is frequently, although by no means predominantly, seen in chronic alcohol abuse. Since heavy drinkers are usually also heavy smokers (the reverse, of course, is not true), the two toxic agents were formerly erroneously incriminated.

History taking should concentrate on alcohol abuse, as should the general and neurologic examination (see Chap. 36). Frequent findings will be a history of numbness of the stocking-and-gloves type, absence of ankle and patellar jerks, and electrophysiological evidence of demyelinating disease, mainly in the spinal cord. This is demonstrated by severe alteration of SSEPs in the presence of normal or near-normal peripheral sensory nerve conduction. Deficient resorption/absorption of B_{12} is demonstrated by blood level and urine excretion tests.

22.2.4 Tumor. Tumors of the anterior fossa may lead to relentless unilateral deterioration of vision. In young individuals this will usually be a *glioma of the optic nerve.* Except for the loss of vision, the history is unremarkable. Frequently, the children do not even complain of headache. Plain x-ray may show enlargement of the optic canal. Neuroimaging permits visualization of the tumor.

In adult patients there are a variety of tumors arising in or extending to the anterior fossa. Frequently, history will reveal a change in personality in addition to the visual symptoms. The patient will have become careless about his job and his family, and will tend to neglect his personal appearance, as well as his areas of interest. His friends may have noticed a loss of initiative and emotional reactions. It is remarkable to what extent these alterations in behavior are tolerated. They rarely prompt a medical examination and frequently are not reported spontaneously, but have to be asked for.

Upon neurologic examination one will find pallor of the optic disc and decreased ipsilateral and contralateral light reaction of the pupil, which typically will react when the sighted eye is illuminated. Another "anterior fossa finding" is unilateral anosmia, which does not alter smell and taste subjectively, but has to be looked for by special examination. EEG, neuroimaging, and angiographical findings will not be discussed here in detail.

23 Muscular Weakness, Proximal

23.1 Myopathy

Bilateral proximal muscular weakness of insidious onset should arouse suspicion primarily of myopathy. In the initial stage of myopathy, weakness disproportionate to the mild degree of muscular atrophy develops. There is no fasciculation of muscle fibers, and reflexes are normal or only slightly attenuated. Of course, there are no paresthesias, nor is there any sensory deficit. The patients may report pain on muscular exercise that suggests widespread affection of the respective muscles, to the extent that the natural alternation between working and resting portions of the muscle(s) no longer functions.

This is clearly seen in electromyography, where the characteristic finding is early recruitment of a great number of muscular fibers, resulting in a very dense pattern of action potentials. Owing to the diseased state of virtually all muscle fibers, the amplitude of the potentials is strikingly small.

Myopathy, of course, is not a precise diagnosis; it merely indicates the diseased organ. Further specification is necessary, because not all myopathies are degenerative in nature. Some are simply one striking feature of a treatable condition, such as metabolic disorder, or autoimmune disease. Family history is usually not very helpful because of the understandable reluctance of the family to reveal the existence of a hereditary disorder.

Laboratory tests may be quite helpful in the identification of a possible underlying cause. The most promising examination is muscle biopsy. Of course, one should ensure that the specimen is seen by a specialist who does not rely only on microscopy and electron microscopy, but will also apply modern enzyme histochemical and immunochemical investigations.

In the scope of this chapter we can only briefly mention the most frequent myopathies; the reader is referred to the textbooks for details. Among the "degenerative" muscular diseases, *muscular dystrophy* should be considered first. The variant which most frequently causes proximal weakness is the "limb girdle" form that is usually first noticed in the 2nd decade of life and takes a relatively benign course. In contrast, the rapidly progressing Duchenne variant, which presents only in 5- to 6-year-old boys, is easily recognized.

The list of nondegenerative myopathies, which is certainly not exhaustive, begins with chronic *thyrotoxic* myopathy. Basically, any *endocrine* disorder may lead to chronic myopathy. Myopathy in *lupus erythematosus* is usually characterized by pain on muscular contraction. *Paraneoplastic* myopathy is frequently present before appearance of the signs and symptoms of the malignancy. "Menopausal myopathy" should be diagnosed only after exclusion of all other causes. Myopathy in disturbances of *glycogen metabolism* occurs mostly in childhood and is characterized by pain on exercise. Generally speaking, painful weakness upon exercise is suggestive of metabolic disease affecting the muscles, and should prompt thorough laboratory investigations and biopsy. It is not a symptom of degenerative muscular disease.

23.2 Polymyositis

In the most common use of the term, polymyositis is an autoimmune disease affecting mainly the muscles of the limbs and pelvic girdle. Age and mode of onset are extremely variable. Characteristic features are bouts and relapses, early appearance of disturbance of swallowing, tenderness of the affected muscles, and laboratory findings suggestive of an acute inflammatory process. Usually, the serum level of creatine kinase is elevated, indicating rapid destruction of muscle fibers. There may be myoglobinuria, which may even lead to acute renal failure by blocking of the tubuli ("crush syndrome"). In children the diagnosis may be facilitated by erythema in the face and on the chest ("dermatomyositis").

EMG shows both "myopathic alteration" as described above, and spontaneous activity indicating damage to the terminal branches of nerves. Biopsy will almost always confirm the diagnosis in the acute stage by showing perivascular and perimysial infiltration by lymphocytes and plasma cells. There may, however, be problems in the chronic stage or during a relapse, where differentiation from muscular dystrophy is sometimes difficult.

Apart from the main group of polymyositis, there are inflammatory processes of muscles owing to recognizable organisms. Examples are myositis of *viral origin*, which has a dramatic onset with severe pain and an extremely fast blood sedimentation rate. Also, circumscribed myositis in sarcoidosis and trichinosis is very painful. The same holds true for *polymyalgia rheumatica*, a very painful muscle disease of the elderly. There is probably little, if any, true muscular weakness, but the severe pain impedes contraction, especially of the muscles of the shoulder and limb girdle. EMG and biopsy do not show affection of muscle fibers. The sedimentation rate is greatly raised, and laboratory parameters suggest subacute inflammatory disease. Some patients eventually develop cranial arteritis (see Chap. 4). The condition responds favorably to immunosuppressive therapy.

23.3 Proximal Diabetic Polyneuropathy

Proximal weakness may also be due to disease of the peripheral nervous system, the most frequent instance being diabetic neuropathy. This common metabolic disorder (see also Chap. 34) has a variant that is not so well known as the standard form with its symmetrical distal sensorimotor signs and symptoms. Some diabetic patients present with proximal weakness in the limb girdle that is usually slightly asymmetrical, frequently painful, but otherwise predominantly motor. The pattern of weakness includes problems in climbing up or down stairs, standing up from the sitting position, and sitting up from the supine position. Ankle jerks may be present, but knee jerks are usually missing, and there is tenderness of the quadriceps muscle.

As in any diabetic affection of peripheral nerves, the metabolic disturbance need not be striking. Sometimes it is recognized only by delayed or incomplete response of the pancreatic beta cells in the glucose tolerance test.

23.4 Neuralgic Amyotrophy

Asymmetrical proximal diabetic polyneuropathy must be distinguished from a unilateral affection of the lumbar plexus that is akin to the well-known neuralgic amyotrophy of the shoulder muscles (see Chap. 24). It has been recognized during the past decade that a similar disease may affect the *lumbar nerve plexus*. The presenting signs and symptoms are those of unilateral acute paralysis of the *femoral nerve*. On close examination, including EMG and nerve conduction studies, one may also find mild affection of neighboring nerves, e.g., of the obturator nerve, leading to weakness of adduction in the hip joint. The condition is benign and will resolve over a period of weeks or months.

It is essential, however, to exclude two conditions requiring special diagnosis and therapy. One is lesion of the *third or fourth lumbar nerve* root, in which case there is no sudomotor paralysis on the anterior aspect of the upper thigh. The autonomic fibers leave the spinal cord no more caudally than with the second lumbar root.

Sudomotor activity *is* paralyzed in *pelvic malignancies*, which invade the lumbar plexus where the autonomic fibers travel to the periphery. Another cause that should be considered is spontaneous hematoma in patients receiving coumarin drugs. Some of them, when they experience the painful beginning of pressure on the femoral nerve, take analgesics that enhance the anticoagulant effect and thus aggravate the hematoma and, consequently, the paralysis.

23.5 Myelitis

Instances of myelitis with proximal paresis have become rare since the virtual elimination of poliomyelitis. Other viral infections, e.g., by coxsackie virus A, may imitate the neurologic syndrome of polio and lead to asymmetrical proximal weakness with areflexia and no sensory disturbance. CSF invariably shows an increase in cell count, mild elevation of the protein level, and a relatively low lactate level.

23.6 Guillain-Barré Syndrome

This type of myelitis should be distinguished from Guillain-Barré syndrome, which is sometimes rather difficult to do during the first few days. The neurologic picture is quite similar: even seventh nerve palsy is seen in both conditions. Nerve conduction studies may be normal during the first few days, and the same holds true for the characteristic elevation of protein in CSF. In case of doubt, pleocytosis speaks in favor of myelitis, although it is also seen in Guillain-Barré syndrome, especially when it has viral etiology, e.g., Epstein-Barr virus. Affection of the autonomic nervous system is a strong point for the diagnosis of Guillain-Barré syndrome only if there is loss of the response of cardiac frequency to vagal nerve stimulation. Bladder dysfunction is seen in both conditions, and the same holds true for respiratory paralysis. Frequently, it is only the course of the disease that permits correct diagnosis on the basis of repeat neurologic examination and nerve conduction studies.

24 Painful States of the Shoulder and Upper Arm

The table preceding this chapter contrasts with the diagnostic monotony encountered in medical practice. All too easily any kind of painful disease state affecting the shoulder and upper arm is given the facile label "shoulder-arm pain" or, even worse, "shoulder-arm syndrome," and automatically subjected to physiotherapy or to intramuscular injections of local anesthetics.

Pain is a symptom that calls for a diagnosis, not a diagnosis in itself. No doctor would seriously consider "abdominal pain" a diagnosis with its own specific set of therapeutic measures. A syndrome is a combination of signs and symptoms; it does not just refer to a particular anatomical region. There is no "hip and leg syndrome," either. Finally, if one does adhere to the mistaken view that in every case pain in the shoulder and arm region is due to mechanical compression of a cervical root by degenerative alteration of the vertebrae or intervertebral discs, it is hard to conceive how this compression could possibly be relieved by the injection of an analgesic drug into any muscle whatever.

These polemic paragraphs are intended to inspire a thoughtful analysis of the patients' signs and symptoms. As in many other diagnostic decisions, consideration of the onset helps to group the pertinent disease states in a preliminary way. Both the acute and the chronic subgroup include malignant and benign diseases.

24.1 Acute Onset

24.1.1 Neuralgic Shoulder Amyotrophy. An acute condition that usually affects the preferred arm, in most cases the right one, neuralgic amyotrophy of the shoulder occurs mainly in young male adults. The presenting symptom is severe pain in the shoulder and upper arm, which may extend along the radial side of the forearm down to the thumb. After several hours, or on the 2nd day, the patient will notice weakness in movements of the shoulder, in addition to his tendency to avoid those movements which aggravate the pain. Movements of the neck do not follow this pattern, which is important for exclusion of a herniated disc.

The extent of weakness can be assessed by the end of the 1st week, when the violent pain has subsided. Examination then reveals affection of the motor fibers of the upper brachial plexus. In most patients there is paresis of the deltoid, serratus anterior, and supraspinatus muscles. The biceps may also be affected. In rare cases, one muscle alone is affected, e.g., the serratus, or the diaphragm. A prominent feature is the rapid onset of muscular atrophy. Reflexes are usually normal, but in some patients there is attenuation of the biceps reflex. Apart from the transient pain there is little, if any, sensory disturbance. This is explained by the fact that the affected part of the plexus carries mostly motor fibers, with the exception of the axillary nerve, of which the area of supply is on the outer surface of the upper arm, but is as small as the palm of the hand.

Nerve conduction studies show slowing of conduction in the brachial plexus, and EMG will reveal denervation of the affected muscles by the end of the 2nd week. CSF is usually normal, and given the characteristic clinical picture, lumbar tap is dispensable. Prognosis is good, but restoration of function may take many months.

24.1.2 Lateral Herniation of a Cervical Disc. By no means abnormal strain is required for the lateral herniation of a cervical disc. The degenerated fibrous ring is very thin, and may burst spontaneously or during such trivial movements as stretching the arm. There is radicular pain. Of greatest diagnostic significance is a fixed position of the head with slight forward inclination and some tilt toward the affected side. Neck movements, in particular reclination, are more painful than arm movements.

Changes in the arm reflexes are usually not very helpful in the acute stage (but see below), and the same holds true for sensory disturbance, given the patient's preoccupation with the acute pain. EMG is normal. X-ray may or may not show degenerative disease of the vertebral column; one need not expect narrowing of the intervertebral distance in all cases. Neuroimaging techniques may show the protrusion of the disc. The important findings are compression of a cervical root in the dorsolateral angle of the cervical channel, or compression of the cord itself. This is recognized by brisker proprioceptive reflexes below the presumed level of damage and by sensory symptoms on the trunk. Some patients present with Brown-Séquard's syndrome (see Chap. 8).

24.1.3 Metastatic Tumor of the Cervical Spine. Acute radicular pain rarely occurs in metastatic tumor of the cervical spine without a fairly long history of premonitory local pain. This, however, is usually erroneously attributed to degenerative vertebral disease (see Sect. 24.1.2).

It is hard, if not impossible, to arrive at the diagnosis on the basis of history and neurologic examination alone. Signs and symptoms are quite similar to those of a herniated disc. A diagnostic clue may be the segmental level, because disc herniation is extremely rare above the level of the sixth cervical root. Laboratory findings may be helpful, but every clinician has seen metastatic tumor with a normal sedimentation rate. Neuroimaging techniques and x-ray are the best methods, followed, if necessary, by myelography, which is conveniently combined with neuroimaging. As long as there is no complete transverse lesion of the spinal cord, one should not lose time searching for a primary malignancy. Surgery may both relieve the cord compression and provide histological findings, but is not, of course, warranted if there is affection of more than one vertebra.

24.1.4 Inflammatory Diseases of the Cervical Spine. Spondylitis has become quite rare. It causes local and referred pain and is recognized by x-ray or neuroimaging techniques. *Intervertebral discitis* may result from operation on a herniated disc. There will be pain upon any movement of the vertebral column, and also referred radicular pain. Neurologic findings are usually unremarkable, except for reflex immobilization of the affected part of the column. Diagnosis rests on radiological examination.

Signs and symptoms in *epidural abscess* are quite dramatic. There is acute onset of unbearable pain, with immobilization of the vertebral column. Signs of spinal cord compression develop rapidly and are considerably more striking than radicular symptoms. There is gross "inflammatory" alteration of laboratory findings, with marked acceleration of sedimentation rate. Neuroimaging techniques are problematic, because the level of lesion is not established on neurologic grounds. The best method is CT myelography, which also provides CSF findings. Cytologic examination may be important in those rare cases where the epidural compression is produced by tumor or lymphoma.

24.1.5 Herpes Zoster. The diagnosis of herpes zoster is difficult, if not impossible, during the first 3–5 days, when there is only radicular pain, prior to the eruption of vesicles within a segmental territory. Usually the pain is of a burning nature, constantly present, and not aggravated by movements or by increase in intraspinal pressure, e.g., by coughing. By the end of the 1st week the diagnosis can be missed only by a doctor who forgoes physical examination. In rare instances there are motor symptoms, such as loss of proprioceptive reflexes and segmental paralyses.

24.1.6 "Frozen Shoulder." The term frozen shoulder usually refers to the final stage of chronically developing disease of the shoulder joint. There are, however, acute exacerbations with acute pain in the shoulder and referred pain in the arm, which force the patient to keep the shoulder joint immobile. Neck movements have little, if any, effect, as does an increase in intraspinal pressure. Abduction of the arm causes both severe pain and reflex contraction of the entire musculature of the shoulder girdle. Motor functions are not testable under these conditions. There is no attenuation of proprioceptive reflexes, or sensory impairment. X-ray shows arthrosis of the shoulder joint and/or calcium deposits in the lateral aspect of the capsule.

24.1.7 "Whiplash Injury." This characteristic trauma to the cervical spine occurs in traffic accidents when a car crashes from behind into another car that is halting or moving slowly. Abrupt acceleration and deceleration of the slower car leads to rapid hyperextension and hyperflexion of the passenger's neck. This results in damage mainly to the intervertebral articulations and ligaments.

With a latency of several hours or a day, nuchal pain develops, forcing the patient to keep his neck immobile and irradiating to the shoulder and upper arm. This painful condition may last several weeks. Reflexes are normal, there is no sensory loss, and electrophysiological and plain x-ray studies are unremarkable. Diagnosis rests on the history. Unfortunately, many patients aggravate their symptoms because they seek financial compensation.

24.2 Chronic Onset

24.2.1 Degenerative Disease of the Cervical Spine. Precisely circumscribed, i.e., monoradicular, pain and sensory disturbances are not usually caused by degenerative disease of the cervical spine. Nor are motor symptoms, i.e., weakness or loss of reflexes, common. The reason is that the symptoms are not, as a rule, due to compression of a nerve root; the pain arises more frequently in the intravertebral joints, which are richly supplied with sensory fibers. Consequently, the symptoms have the character of referred pain, which is rather diffuse and is not accompanied by segmental sensory or motor loss. Movements of the neck are limited, but do not necessarily provoke bouts of pain. Shoulder movements are not restricted as long as there is no secondary shrinkage of the capsule owing to immobilization of the arm.

24.2.2 Extramedullary Tumor of the Cervical Spinal Cord. In contrast, extramedullary tumor is likely to damage the pertinent nerve root fairly early, especially since more than half of these tumors are neuromas that arise from a dorsal root. Moreover, meningioma is usually located on the dorsal aspect of the cord. There is radicular pain, aggravated by coughing. Early in the course of the disease radicular sensory loss, and frequently alterations in reflexes, occur. It is important to recognize affection of one or two nerve roots, because diagnosis should be achieved prior to damage to the cord itself, which might be irreversible. Electrophysiological studies require a great deal of skill and experience. Plain x-ray is quite often unremarkable; neuroimaging techniques and CT myelography are needed.

24.2.3 Pancoast's Tumor. The clinical picture and course of events in Pancoast's tumor are described in detail in Chap. 17. Suffice it here to mention that pain in the area of supply of the lower brachial plexus, i.e., along the ulnar aspect of the arm and hand, arises rather late in the development of the tumor. If there is ipsilateral Horner's syndrome there is virtually no diagnostic alternative, except for syringomyelia.

24.2.4 Syringomyelia and Intramedullary Tumor. Since the cavity within the spinal cord exerts pressure on both the lateral horn, i.e., the central sympathetic pathway, and the posterior horn, i.e., the area of segmental sensory influx into the cord, the initial symptom may be radicular pain. Usually this is not precisely confined to one or two segments, but is diffused over the arm. At this stage there may be central Horner's syndrome and sudomotor paralysis in the ipsilateral face, shoulder, and arm (see Chap. 17). This combination of signs and symptoms indicates chronic disease within the cord itself.

The alternative to syringomyelia is intramedullary tumor, which, for all practical purposes, will be benign. Early recognition is mandatory, because in both instances damage to the cord will be irreversible if diagnosis is made only after the occurrence of segmental muscular atrophy owing to anterior horn lesion, spastic paraplegia owing to pyramidal tract damage, or a transverse syndrome with specific loss of awareness of pain and temperature. Neuroimaging techniques are mandatory, preferably in combination with myelography.

96

24.2.5 Arthrosis of the Shoulder Joint. It should be mentioned briefly that arthrosis of the shoulder joint may cause referred pain in the arm, with no sensory or motor deficit. The prominent feature is progressive immobilization of the shoulder with pain caused by abduction of the arm.

24.2.6 Thoracic Outlet Syndrome. The thoracic outlet syndrome is discussed in Chap. 27. It is a cause of radicular pain that is not easily recognized.

24.2.7 Postherpetic Neuralgia. As a rule, neuralgia following herpes zoster is attributed to degenerative disease of the vertebral column, because most if not all of the patients are of advanced age, and frequently radiography is performed prior to instead of after physical examination. The pain is much more agonizing than in vertebral arthrosis and is not influenced by movement or by coughing. Usually the sequelae of the zoster vesicles can be seen as brownish spots in segmental distribution.

24.2.8 Regional Psychogenic Pain. Last, but not least, the correct diagnosis may be regional psychogenic pain. This condition is frequent, but the diagnosis should be made with caution, as in all psychogenic painful states. The fact that neurologic and ancillary examinations are unremarkable does not preclude the presence of unrecognized disease. So, again, the advice is to meet these patients with an encouraging attitude, to give them antidepressant drugs, most of which have an analgesic side effect, but not to forget repeat control examinations.

25 Paraplegia of Chronic Evolution

Patients with this condition present with or without sensory symptoms and/or disturbances of micturition. Sensory symptoms may occur as numbness, spontaneous tingling sensations, or pain. The distribution of these sensations is most frequently of the stocking type, slowly ascending and eventually covering the lower part of the body. Pain usually has a segmental distribution and indicates the level of a spinal cord lesion. In these instances it increases when the patient coughs or presses for defecation. Finally, there is a rare but very important symptom consisting of paresthesias running down the patient's back or along the arms with a proximal to distal distribution, which is referred to as Lhermitte's sign. It is indicative of an inflammatory, neoplastic or traumatic lesion at the level of the cervical portion of the spinal cord. Disorders of micturition are either incontinence or retention.

All these symptoms can be assessed in a short interview. Furthermore, observation of the patient's gait upon entering the consultation room frequently permits the distinction between a peripheral (bilateral footdrop) and a central (increased extensor tone wih bilateral circumduction) paraparesis. Thus, a hypothesis as to the level of the lesion(s) and to the extension within the spinal cord can be made before starting the neurologic examination.

Unfortunately, most patients with spastic paraplegia of chronic evolution are misdiagnosed as having degenerative disease of the lower lumbar vertebrae and/or a herniated lumbar disc. Very rarely do we see a patient with central paraparesis who has not received extensive x-ray examinations of the lumbar portion of the vertebral column, including spinal neuroimaging, although for anatomical reasons lesions at that level can cause only peripheral, not central, paresis.

There are roughly ten conditions that must be considered in these patients, and their description makes it clear that there is no possibility of a quick diagnosis.

25.1 Spinal Tumor and Spinal Angioma

Although spinal tumors are rare (their frequency is one-seventh of that of brain tumors), the diagnosis is of the utmost importance, because most of them are histologically benign and can be completely removed if recognized early enough, whereas they lead to irreversible damage of the spinal cord if early diagnosis is missed. The leading symptoms are a relentlessly progressive course; affection of all systems of the cord – motor, sensory, and autonomic; absence of signs and symptoms above a certain segmental level; and segmental pain of girdle distribution, especially when intraspinal pressure is raised, e.g., by coughing.

Spinal angioma is conspicuous by its fluctuating symptoms, and disturbances of micturition are experienced at an early stage. Spinal arteriovenous fistula, on the other hand, located chiefly at the thoracic level, has a chronic progressive course and occurs in the 50- to 60-year-old age group.

Because of the eccentric localization of the long pathways within the spinal cord, neurologic examination is likely to suggest that the lesion is located at a lower level than it really is. Consequently, spinal neuroimaging focussed on that level may give a false-negative result. Comparison of somatosensory evoked potentials (SSEPs) after stimulation of the tibial and median nerve and dermatome evoked potentials (DEPs) sometimes permits a crude localization.

My personal preference, therefore, is for myelography, which can be done quickly and safely, and permits in most instances a clear diagnosis. It also provides CSF findings. Incidentally, it can be combined with spinal neuroimaging examination focussed on the locus of lesion, with a view to demonstrating possible extraspinal portions of a tumor.

25.2 Multiple Sclerosis

A diagnosis of multiple sclerosis of spinal localization is tenuous, and should be questioned repeatedly. It is true that there is a certain connection between advanced age at onset and predominantly spinal localization of the lesions. It is equally true, however, that careful history taking frequently reveals bouts and relapses. Lhermitte's sign is frequently positive, but is not diagnostic of multiple sclerosis. Also, examination of visual, somatosensory, and auditory evoked potentials, together with the blink reflex, is likely to demonstrate supraspinal lesions. Neuroimaging shows both, areas of hypodensity that do not correspond to vascular territories and, frequently, global reduction of brain volume. Should these ancillary examinations not demonstrate "multiplicity in space," and should history not suggest "multiplicity in time," then examination of CSF is warranted with a view to demonstrating the presence of plasma cells and/or production of IgG within the CNS. The danger of missing a spinal tumor cannot be overestimated.

25.3 Combined Degeneration of the Spinal Cord

For a long period, combined degeneration of the spinal cord is characterized by central motor and sensory symptoms with no pain. Bladder dysfunction occurs only at a very advanced stage of the disease. The combination of signs and symptoms does not suggest a distinct localization within the spinal cord, thus producing some resemblance to multiple sclerosis. There are, however, no bouts and relapses, Lhermitte's sign is negative, and supraspinal symptoms occur only at a very late stage. Diagnosis is made by demonstration of deficient intestinal uptake, and lowered serum level, of vitamin B_{12}.

25.4 Cervical Spondylotic Myelopathy

In the presence of a particularly narrow spinal canal and protruded discs, cervical myelopathy may occur. There is no massive herniation; consequently, the findings call for a very critical evaluation of the mechanical (and vascular) factors that produce progressive damage to the cervical cord. Myelography with different degrees of inclination and reclination of the head is mandatory. The decision to perform laminectomy is difficult to take.

25.5 Radiation Myelopathy

The diagnosis of radiation myelopathy is made entirely on clinical grounds. It is most frequently seen in patients with lymphoma at the cervical or upper thoracic level. The patients present with a progressive transverse lesion of the spinal cord with leading sensory symptoms, such as paresthesias and pain.

A history of radiation treatment should arouse suspicion and prevent confusion with an intraspinal malignancy which would call for further radiation treatment. Neuroimaging and myelography are not reliably diagnostic one way or the other, nor is cytologic examination of CSF, because the malignancy may grow in the subdural space, whereas radiation myelopathy does not necessarily lead to abnormal CSF findings.

25.6 Motor Neuron Disease

The onset of motor neuron disease may be marked by spastic paraparesis and it may thus bear a superficial resemblance to a spinal cord tumor. There are, however, no sensory symptoms, no pain, and no bladder dysfunction. On the other hand, careful examination may reveal early signs of chronic denervation, such as muscular fasciculation or atrophy. Generalized denervation can often be demonstrated earlier by EMG than by inspection. Denervation in the presence of increased reflexes is diagnostic, provided there are no sensory symptoms. Equally diagnostic is an increased or even clonic jaw reflex, which is seen only in motor neuron disease, in arteriosclerotic pseudobulbar paralysis, and in tetanus, and these three conditions cannot seriously be confused. In case of doubt, biopsy of the sural nerve is helpful, because, as a rule, a sensory nerve should not be affected in motor neuron disease.

25.7 Syringomyelia

For syringomyelia see Chap. 27.

25.8 Disease Processes of the Cervicocranial Junction

Only brief mention is made of disease processes at the cervicocranial junction. The diagnosis is made on radiological grounds, and the task of the doctor is to ask for x-ray or neuroimaging examination at a sufficiently high level.

25.9 Chronic Vascular Myelopathy

In my view, chronic vascular myelopathy is a diagnosis which is impossible to verify in vivo unless it is caused by venous obstruction, e.g., in cases of an arteriovenous fistula, which can be identified by myelography and spinal angiography.

26 Progressive Clouding of Consciousness

All conditions listed in the table are described extensively in other chapters. In order to avoid duplications, this chapter will be kept short and the reader is referred to the index for details, but it appears essential to discuss briefly a group of disease states that may be a diagnostic challenge both to the family doctor and to the house doctor on the emergency ward.

26.1 Intoxication

Certainly, the main reason for progressive clouding of consciousness is intoxication. Progression, therefore, is due to advancing absorption of the drug. Oculomotor dysfunction corresponds to the level of vigilance, and there may be slow spontaneous bilateral horizontal deviations, conjugate or disconjugate. The oculocephalic reflex, i.e., reflex movements of the eyes in the opposite direction upon labyrinthine stimulation when the doctor moves the patient's head in the lateral or vertical plane, may be absent. There may be no ocular responses to caloric stimulation. Pupils become small and are still reactive, but with progression of coma they dilate, and reaction to light is lost. The limbs may show decerebrate rigidity; later on they become flaccid.

The diagnosis of intoxication cannot be made without ancillary examinations. Neuroimaging is normal, as are CW ultrasound findings. EEG shows predominant beta activity after ingestion of barbiturates and benzodiazepines. There is generalized abnormality with other drugs. Electrophysiological studies show only cortical and brain stem dysfunction. Blood and urine tests are required, and forced diuresis is applied, provided there is sufficient reason for assuming intoxication.

26.2 Space-Occupying Intracranial Lesion

A space-occupying intracranial lesion (tumor, hematoma, abscess) is suspected if there are signs of focal brain damage. The reason for rapid deterioration may be rupture of one of the vessels feeding the tumor or an increase in brain edema which is mostly due to interference with venous drainage. History may be unremarkable, and papilledema need not be present. EEG will show focal and generalized dysfunction. Performing a lumbar tap is hazardous: it may lead to temporal lobe or cerebellar herniation with compression of the brain stem. Neuro-imaging techniques or cerebral angiography will provide the diagnosis.

26.3 Thrombosis of Intracerebral Sinus(es)

Rarely is progressive clouding of consciousness the only sign of thrombosis of intracerebral sinus(es). In most instances, the first signs are epileptic fits and mono- or hemiparesis. If these are observed in childbed, the diagnosis is probably venous thrombosis. There are, however, many instances of "spontaneous" thrombosis where no immediate clues are available. Lumbar tap may show pleocytosis with presence of erythrocytes. Diagnosis rests on neuroimaging or angiography, with special attention to speed of flow and visualization of the sinuses during the late phase. Once diagnosis is established, a thorough hemostasiological investigation is mandatory.

26.4 Encephalitis

The diagnosis of encephalitis is discussed in Chap. 3. It is important to note that there are two variants. Postinfectious, perivenous encephalitis leads primarily to signs and symptoms of diffuse brain disease. The most prominent of these are decrease in vigilance, generalized epileptic seizures, and generalized slowing of the EEG traces with slight, if any, focal signs. In contrast, invasion of the brain tissue by viruses will cause focal damage to one of the hemispheres, e.g., aphasia or hemiplegia, in addition to progressive clouding of consciousness.

26.5 Wernicke's Encephalopathy

The early appearance of pupillary signs, such as dilated pupils of unequal size with impaired reaction to light, should facilitate recognition of Wernicke's encephalopathy (see Chaps. 10 and 20). These signs are due to midbrain damage. At that stage, consciousness will be only mildly impaired, because the reticular activating system is not yet severely affected. Very few patients do not present with signs of chronic alcohol abuse, such as slight jaundice, ectatic veins, tremor of the outstretched hands, and loss of ankle jerks.

26.6 Status Epilepticus (Petit Mal – Complex Partial Seizures)

An uninterrupted sequence of petit mal or complex partial seizures does not lead to *progressive* clouding of consciousness. It is discussed here because the sudden onset of impairment of vigilance may have escaped attention. Very rarely is status epilepticus the first sign of epileptic disease, but if the patient is known to be epileptic, diagnosis should be easy. The leading symptoms are motor stereotypes. In the case of petit mal status these are nystactic upward movements of the eyes with a frequency of roughly 3/s, and, sometimes, twitching of the facial muscles. In complex partial seizures there are the well-known chewing or swallowing movements and/or all kinds of stereotyped actions involving both hands, and sometimes also vocalization. The suspicion is confirmed by EEG, which shows either uninterrupted trains of generalized spikes and waves with a frequency of 3/s, or bilateral slow and sharp waves over the temporal leads.

26.7 Metabolic Derangement

Signs and symptoms of metabolic derangement are quite unspecific, and recognition is possible only on the basis of extensive laboratory investigations. The most frequent condition is hyperglycemia, especially the nonketotic hyperosmolar variant.

26.8 Blood Hyperviscosity

Not infrequently, elderly patients who are not adequately taken care of arrive at a stage of progressive clouding of consciousness because of blood hyperviscosity. This does not happen only in the patient's home, where he simply forgets to drink; the neurologic consultant will also be called to see patients in the surgical department who are postoperatively supplied intravenously with an insufficient amount of fluid.

27 Progressive Wasting of Hand Muscles

The differential diagnosis of progressive wasting of distal hand muscles is facilitated by three preliminary considerations:

- Are signs and symptoms confined to the upper extremities, or is there indication by neurologic findings or electromyography or nerve conduction studies that the legs are also affected? If they are, the patient has polyneuropathy, motor neuron disease, or myopathy, in that order of frequency (see Chap. 25). If they are not, the following questions are suggested:
- Are signs and symptoms unilateral or bilateral? Unilateral affections, as a rule, are suggestive of treatable conditions. Bilateralism is strongly suggestive of systemic disease of the spinal cord or of the musculature.
- Are signs and symptoms strictly motor or sensorimotor? Absence of sensory disturbances has an ominous prognostic meaning. Presence of sensory signs and symptoms helps to pinpoint the locus of lesion.

27.1 Unilateral

27.1.1 Carpal Tunnel Syndrome (Median Nerve Entrapment Syndrome). Distal entrapment of the median nerve under the transverse carpal ligament causes carpal tunnel syndrome. The patients first experience sensory symptoms, i.e., numbness or pinprick paresthesias on the volar aspect of the tumb and the index and middle fingers, especially in the night and during daytime rest. In the initial stage these symptoms are alleviated by shaking motions of the hand. If the correct diagnosis is missed, progressive wasting of the abductor and opponens pollicis muscles ensues, while all other muscles of the hand that are supplied by the ulnar, and to a very limited extent by the radial, nerve remain

105

intact. The function of the two muscles is easily tested. The abductor brevis muscle moves the thumb in a plane 90° relative to the palm of the hand. Weakness of the muscle prevents the patient from grasping an object, which is conveniently tested with a water glass. In order to test the opposition action of the thumb, the patient holds the hand palm up with outstretched fingers and is asked to approximate the little finger with the thumb in a rotating movement. History and findings are quite characteristic.

Nerve conduction study has three purposes: to verify the diagnosis, to establish the degree of damage to the nerve for follow-up after operation, and to find out if there are also signs of polyneuropathy, i.e., of generalized disease of the peripheral nervous system. "Latent" polyneuropathy not infrequently produces a predisposition to entrapment syndromes. If present, it requires additional diagnostic measures and therapy.

27.1.2 Ulnar Nerve Paralysis. The most frequent peripheral nerve palsy is ulnar nerve paralysis. Damage to the nerve occurs either at the elbow or wrist joint. Acute traumatic lesions should pose no diagnostic problems. We are concerned here with chronic damage of insidious onset.

Since the ulnar nerve innervates most of the intrinsic hand muscles, the patient, as well as the doctor, might suspect that this is a case of motor neuron disease. This diagnosis is ruled out if sensory disturbance is present in the area of supply of the superficial branch of the nerve, i.e., on the volar and dorsal aspect of the fourth and little fingers and the adjacent area of the hand. Sensory disturbance in ulnar nerve palsy does not extend to the entire forearm. If it does, one has to consider damage to the brachial plexus or a radicular lesion at the level of the seventh or eighth cervical root.

Motor symptoms, i.e., weakness and wasting, are to be analyzed with equal care. Are they limited to the muscles supplied by the ulnar nerve? In other words, is the thenar, which is for all practical purposes innervated solely by the median nerve, spared? If this is the case, one may proceed to establishing the locus of lesion, which also gives some hints as to etiology.

The most common site of damage to the ulnar nerve is at the elbow. There are sensory as well as motor signs and symptoms, and atrophy is seen in the interosseus muscles and in the hypothenar. In full-blown ulnar palsy the patient presents with the so-called claw hand, characterized by hyperextension in the metacarpophalangeal joints and flexion in the interphalangeal joints. This is most striking in the fourth and little fingers. There is paralysis of abduction and adduction of the fingers. Failure of adduction of the thumb is demonstrated by making the patient take a notebook or a spatula with both hands

106

between thumb and index finger and asking him to attempt to tear it apart. He will then compensate for the weak adductor pollicis muscle by flexing the thumb in the interphalangeal joints, which is a median nerve function.

The ulnar nerve is damaged at the elbow following local trauma, sometimes with a latency of many years; by degenerative disease of the joint; by straining the nerve in occupations that require very frequent flexion and extension of the forearm; and, last but not least, by pressure in bedridden patients.

Less common, and sometimes difficult to recognize, are the sequelae of damage to the nerve at the wrist joint. In these cases sensory disturbance may be absent or limited to the volar aspect of the hand, because the sensory branches leave the nerve proximal to the wrist. Flexion of the hand is completely preserved, because the flexor carpi ulnaris muscle at the forearm is not denervated. In many instances there is a striking difference between the atrophic dorsal interosseus muscle between thumb and index finger and the relatively or completely spared hypothenar. This type of lesion is caused by local trauma, pressure (e.g., in cyclists), or degenerative disease of the wrist joint.

27.1.3 Pancoast's Tumor. The early symptoms of Pancoast's tumor are described in Chap. 17. Wasting of hand muscles occurs long after ipsilateral miosis and attenuation of sweating have indicated affection of the cervical sympathetic chain. When the cancer invades the lower portions of the brachial plexus, the patient suffers continuous pain, which is localized first in the axilla and which then extends along the ulnar side of the arm down to the hand. All too often, any kind of referred pain is attributed to degenerative disease of the vertebral column, and this is true even when wasting of hand muscles ensues. This misdiagnosis is particularly unfortunate, because once invasion of the brachial plexus has occurred, chances of successful surgical treatment are nil, and furthermore radiotherapy will bear the risk of additional damage to the plexus.

27.1.4 Thoracic Outlet Syndrome. Wasting of hand muscles is a late sign also in thoracic outlet syndrome, and the diagnosis should have been made long before its appearance. The syndrome is caused by compression of the brachial plexus and the subclavian artery between the medial and anterior scalene muscles, both of which insert on the ventral portion of the first rib. Normally, this interstice, which is called the scalene groove, leaves sufficient space, whether the arm is elevated or pulled down by carrying a heavy load. In some persons, however a cervical rib, a fibrous ligament, or an abnormally large insertion of the medial scalene muscle leads to narrowing of the scalene groove and, consequently, to entrapment that is initially caused by extreme positions of the arm and later becomes chronic. The diagnosis requires demonstration of both damage to the lower brachial plexus and compression of the subclavian artery. The latter is done by Adson's maneuvre, in which the patient is asked to turn his head toward the side of the suspected lesion, to recline the head, and to perform a deep inspiration. These movements narrow the scalene groove and lead to attenuation of flow in the subclavian artery, which can be palpated at the radial artery and objectively measured by CW ultrasound sonography.

27.1.5 Motor Neuron Disease. Sometimes, motor neuron disease starts unilaterally with wasting of hand muscles. There is no pain or any other sensory disturbance, neither is there pupillary or sudomotor abnormality. The diagnosis is discussed in the next paragraph.

27.2 Bilateral

27.2.1 Motor Neuron Disease. By far the most frequent cause of bilateral wasting of the hand muscles is motor neuron disease (see also Sect. 27.1.5). In many patients, there is both wasting and increase of tendon reflexes in the same limb, indicating affection of the central motor pathways and the anterior horn. In the absence of sensory signs and symptoms, this syndrome leaves no diagnostic alternative. A useful sign corroborating the diagnosis is the spontaneous fasciculation of muscle fibers characteristic of chronic denervation. Denervation can frequently be demonstrated by electromyography also in apparently unaffected muscles. Sometimes the serum level of creatine kinase is elevated. In case of doubt, biopsy of the sural nerve, which is a purely sensory branch of the peroneal nerve should be performed. The sural nerve should, of course, be patent in motor neuron disease.

In most instances the disease has no recognizable cause. Yet, given the lack of an effective therapy and the fatal outcome of the disease after a maximum duration of 10 years, a search for a malignancy should be conducted, because there are rare cases of paraneoplastic degeneration of the "pyramidal" motor system. Also, syphilitic disease should be ruled out.

27.2.2 Progressive Anterior Horn Degeneration. Progressive degeneration of the anterior horn (spinal muscular atrophy of the Aran-Duchenne type) is a very rare disease that bears some resemblance to motor neuron disease. Initially, there is wasting and, to a lesser degree, weakness of hand muscles with fasciculation and no sensory disturbance. Signs of pyramidal tract involvement are lacking, however, and the progression of the disease is very slow. In contrast to motor neuron disease the patients do not, as a rule, develop bulbar palsy.

27.2.3 Hereditary Distal Muscular Dystrophy. A rare distal myopathy may imitate anterior horn cell degeneration. The diagnosis of hereditary distal myopathy rests on electromyography and muscle biopsy. It is important to recognize the myopathic nature of the disease, because progression is slow and rarely do patients become severely incapacitated.

28 Ptosis of the Upper Eyelid

Ptosis has one of three causes: partial damage to the oculomotor nerve (the branch which innervates the levator palpebrae superioris muscle); damage to the sympathetic pathway (weakness of tarsal muscle; see also Chap. 17); or myopathy. Ptosis may be unilateral or bilateral. If it is unilateral, it indicates a circumscribed lesion. Bilateral ptosis is almost invariably a sign of generalized muscle disease or, much more rarely, of disease of the peripheral nervous system. The first diagnostic task is to ascertain whether there is also mild weakness in other extraocular muscles, and the second is to examine the pupil(s) for width and reaction to light. Presence of miosis and preservation of ocular movement suggest Horner's syndrome and rule out third nerve palsy. A mildly dilated pupil with attenuation of ipsilateral constriction reaction to light is characteristic of third nerve palsy and rules out both Horner's syndrome and myopathy. There are, of course, cases of third nerve palsy where the parasympathetic fibers are spared. For differential diagnosis of third nerve palsy, see Chap. 6. In myopathy, there is frequently weakness of other ocular, facial, and/or limb muscles, in addition to ptosis.

Quite naturally, there is a great deal of overlap between this chapter and the one on acute paralysis of the extraocular muscles. Some of the following paragraphs, therefore, may be kept rather short. They should serve simply as a reminder, because ptosis may be an accidental finding, and it rarely leads to complaints by the patient. If it evolves chronically, some patients cannot even tell whether or not they have had a drooping of the eyelid(s) all their life.

28.1 Unilateral

28.1.1 Horner's Syndrome. The differential diagnosis of Horner's syndrome is discussed in Chap. 17.

28.1.2 Lesion of the Midbrain Tegmentum. A midbrain tegmentum lesion which, within the complex of the third nerve nucleus, affects only the small area where the fibers to the levator palpebrae superioris muscle originate, must be very small indeed. It is observed, however, in small-vessel disease of the brain stem. Usually, the patients are hypertensive. Metastatic midbrain tumor will rapidly produce other local signs in addition to ptosis of the upper eye lid.

The midbrain lacune itself will be smaller than the resolving power of modern imaging machines. However, if one suspects stenosing small-artery disease it is useful to search, by neuroimaging, for the presence of other lacunes that would support the diagnosis.

28.1.3 Syndrome of the Cavernous Sinus. The cavernous sinus syndrome has been discussed in Chap. 21. Unilateral ptosis may be the first sign of a fistula between the carotid artery and the cavernous sinus. These fistulae sometimes develop spontaneously, most probably by rupture of a small arteriosclerotic aneurysm, and this is by no means a dramatic event. In our experience, fluctuation in the intensity of ptosis is quite suggestive, and CW ultrasound sonography may be diagnostic, as described in Chap. 6.

Any kind of parasellar tumor should be considered, especially if in addition to ptosis there is pain in the ocular or temporal region, and if there is slight protrusion of the eyeball and/or congestion of conjunctival vessels.

28.1.4 Intraorbital Tumor and Inflammatory Pseudotumor. If intraorbital tumor leads to drooping of the upper eye lid, the mechanism is damage to one of the terminal branches of the third nerve. Otherwise, tumor and retro-orbital inflammatory processes of various types lead rather to widening of the eyelids. Frequently there is nonpulsating protrusion of the eyeball, which can be assessed by comparing the position of two spatulae placed horizontally on the eyes, lids closed. Diagnosis is made by neuroimaging and the nature of the process may be verified by biopsy.

28.2 Bilateral

28.2.1 Myopathy. The most frequent cause is myopathy. Onset in these cases is insidious, and close examination will reveal signs of atrophy in other muscles of the face, which give the patient a slack expression devoid of the normal fast succession of emotional facial movement(s) (so-called myopathic facies). In addition to ptosis there may be weakness of the ring muscles of the eyes and mouth, and weakness of proximal limb muscles. As progression is quite slow in this group of diseases, the patients develop strategies of innervation by which they compensate for the weakness, of which they are not fully aware.

The rare *myopathies in childhood* will not be discussed here, particularly since ptosis in these children is not the presenting sign.

The onset of *Steinert's disease* (dystrophia myotonica) occurs in early adulthood. The half-closed eyes give the patient a sleepy expression that is underscored by the inadequacy of his efforts to conceal his condition. Incidentally, many of these patients are in fact rather slow in mentation. The dystrophic process eventually affects all muscles, particularly the sternomastoid, brachioradial, and peroneal muscles. Consequently, many patients have bilateral footdrop (see also Chap. 15). Demonstration of percussion myotonia, myotonic discharges in the electromyogram, cataracts and cardiomyopathy, to name but a few of the prominent features, facilitates the diagnosis.

Some of the variants of *progressive muscular dystrophy* may start between the ages of 20 and 30 with bilateral ptosis. Sooner or later there will also be weakness in the extraocular muscles. Owing to the slow progression of the disease, diplopia is not usually present. Rather, the patients suppress visual information from one eye. It is characteristic of this group of diseases that the patients try to compensate for the ptosis by reclining the head and continuously innervating the frontalis muscle (i.e., lifting the eyebrows) which gives the face an expression of surprise.

28.2.2 Ophthalmoplegia Plus. Progressive external ophthalmoplegia is a group of degenerative diseases, the most puzzling of which has been termed Kearns-Sayre syndrome or, more conveniently, ophthalmoplegia plus. Bilateral ptosis and affection of extraocular muscles without diplopia occur, but there are also signs of involvement of the CNS, such as cerebellar ataxia and spastic paraparesis. Some patients are demented, others deaf. Some have pigment degeneration of the retina. Onset is in early adulthood, the course is slowly progressive, and there is no therapy.

28.2.3 Myasthenia Gravis. Unilateral or bilateral ptosis may herald myasthenia gravis, which is extensively discussed in Chap. 40. The patient's chief complaint is drooping of the eyelids in the course of the day, in particular during prolonged "intentional" visual activity such as reading, driving, or watching television. At the examination, ptosis becomes evident after repeated innervation of the levator palpebrae superioris muscle, e.g., by making the patient open the eyelids as forcefully as possible, preferably in a supine position. In many, but unfortunately not in all cases, the weakness can be reversed by intravenous injection of edrophonium hydrochloride, which acts on the postsynaptic membrane and thus overcomes the myasthenic deficit in presynaptic acetylcholine. If this is a case of ocular myasthenia without weakness of other extraocular muscles, EMG with stimulation of a peripheral nerve is likely to be negative, as will be the search for antibodies against acetylcholine receptors or skeletal muscles.

28.2.4 Lesion of the Midbrain Tegmentum. More extensive, i.e., bilateral, lesions of the Midbrain Tegmentum may give rise to bilateral ptosis (see also Sect. 28. 1.2).

28.2.5 Hereditary Metabolic Neuropathy. Ptosis may be the presenting sign in rare hereditary metabolic neuropathies, such as Refsum's syndrome or Bassen-Kornzweig syndrome. Absence of proprioceptive reflexes and slowing of nerve conduction will indicate disease of the peripheral nervous system. The youth of the patient should prompt a search for metabolic deficiency.

28.2.6 Blepharospasm. Ptosis is not infrequently confused with closure of the eyes by spasmodic innervation of the orbicularis oculi muscles. The condition is called blepharospasm, but this is a purely descriptive term with no explanatory value. In some cases the hyperkinesia heralds Huntington's disease. This suspicion can be corroborated by a positive family history. Unfortunately this is rarely obtained, because the family prefers to obscure the existence of a hereditary condition. Further important features are involuntary movements in the fingers or toes.

Blepharospasm may be accompanied by hyperkinesia solely in midline muscles, in particular those of the face and the respiratory/phonatory apparatus. In addition to spasmodic closure of the eyes, the patient may be conspicuous by irregular respiration and a squeaky voice. The condition is called Meige's syndrome, but its neurologic status has not yet been firmly established.

Finally, blepharospasm may be psychogenic. This is a very problematic diagnosis and is probably frequently erroneous. At any rate, the patient should be regularly reexamined for other signs of extrapyramidal disorder.

29 Pupillary Abnormality Plus Areflexia

29.1   Adie's Syndrome
29.2   Tabes Dorsalis
29.3   Diabetic Polyneuropathy
29.4   Combined Degeneration of the Spinal Cord

If the pupils are abnormal in width, form, reaction to light, and accommodation/near sight, and if in addition proprioceptive reflexes, at least ankle jerks, are absent, many doctors will suspect syphilitic disease of the nervous system. There are, however, at least three other conditions to be considered.

29.1 Adie's Syndrome

Fully developed Adie's syndrome consists of moderately dilated pupils that apparently do not react to light or to accommodation/near sight, and of absent ankle jerks. Sometimes the knee jerks are also missing, and in rare cases there is complete areflexia. Sensory functions are normal, as is motor and sensory nerve conduction. The patient complains of being dazzled by bright light or by the sun, and of experiencing difficulty in focussing on small objects at close range. On superficial examination the pupils do not show phasic constriction on illumination or on accommodation/near sight. In Chap. 34, methods of observing tonic constriction and dilation are described. In addition, a simple pharmacologic test is given, which demonstrates parasympathetic denervation hypersensitivity of the affected sphincter muscle of the iris.

History is very revealing. Most patients have noticed one morning that one of their pupils is wider than its companion. At the same time they noticed accommodation problems and hypersensitivity to bright light. At that stage reflexes may still be patent. Over many years, areflexia very slowly develops, and eventually the second eye is also affected.

One hesitates to call the condition a disease. Apart from the symptoms described, it causes no harm, and there are no other signs or symptoms. Adie's syndrome requires no treatment except the suggestion that sunglasses should be worn. The greatest problem is to prevent the doctor from performing a lumbar tap with the intention of demonstrating tabes dorsalis. Syphilitic affection is ruled out by normal serological reactions in venous blood.

29.2 Tabes Dorsalis

On the other hand, in tabes dorsalis the affected pupil is smaller than normal and not quite circular, and while it does not react to light at all, reaction to accommodation/near sight is prompt and full (Argyll Robertson pupil). In further contrast to Adie's syndrome, both eyes are usually affected at the beginning. Areflexia is accompanied by a variety of sensory symptoms, ranging from impairment of postural sensibility, which leads to locomotor ataxia when visual control of movements is prevented by closure of the eyes, to impairment in the appreciation of vibration and spontaneous circumscribed pain. On the other hand, painful stimuli are quite often felt only with a considerable delay. Nerve conduction studies are normal. It is beyond the scope of this book to describe the full syndrome of tabes dorsalis in detail, because once the patient has reached an advanced stage there will be no difficulty with differential diagnosis.

29.3 Diabetic Polyneuropathy

Certainly, the most frequent disease of the peripheral nervous system is diabetic polyneuropathy. Absence of ankle jerks and attenuation of vibration sensation are very common even in patients who have no complaints about their motor or sensory functions. Quite often, the autonomic nervous system is also involved, and a very common sign is narrowing of the pupils with slow and incomplete reaction to light and to accommodation/near sight, which permits distinction from Argyll Robertson pupil. Nerve conduction studies are always pathologic and show slowing of motor and/or sensory conduction velocity. Evoked potentials are affected only to the degree of affection of the peripheral nerves.

29.4 Combined Degeneration of the Spinal Cord

A protean combination of signs and symptoms marks combined degeneration of the spinal cord. For this discussion, the most important patients are the roughly 50% who present with absent ankle jerks. Paresthesia and disturbance of those sensory qualities that are mediated by the posterior columns are regular complaints. Not infrequently, both pupils are small, but their reactions are normal. Nerve conduction studies show slowing of motor and sensory conduction velocity. Due to affection of the posterior column, sensory evoked potentials are altered over and above the degree attributable to the peripheral dam-

115

age. This holds true in particular for potentials evoked from the tibial and sural nerves. Serological reactions for syphilis are, of course, negative.

The diagnosis is easy when plantar extensor signs develop; these are seen in about 50% of cases. Obviously, one has to demonstrate impaired intestinal absorption of vitamin B_{12}.

30 Sensory Disturbance of the Tongue

30.1 Unilateral (Affection of the Lingual Nerve)

Sensory disturbance in one half of the tongue indicates an affection of the lingual nerve, which is one of the major sensory branches of the mandibular nerve, the third branch of the trigeminal nerve. The lingual nerve innervates the anterior two-thirds of the tongue, yet quite frequently the patient is not spontaneously aware that the posterior third of the tongue, supplied by the glossopharyngeal nerve, is spared. Even on examination he may venture that sensation is altered over the entire surface of the tongue. One cannot expect an anatomically naive person to subjectively elaborate and respect the niceties of neuroanatomy.

The patient may feel numbness or pain, or both. Pain does not usually have the characteristic features of trigeminal neuralgia ("tic douloureux"), but either is constantly present or waxes and wanes over longer periods. As a rule, it is not triggered by sensory stimulation or movement. The pain quite frequently has a burning quality. Some patients experience a decrease in the sense of taste and some do not. After all, sensation on the other half of the tongue and in the mucosa of the oral cavity is preserved.

It is important to establish that the sensory disturbance is limited to the tongue and does not extend to the area of supply of the inferior alveolar nerve. This area includes the teeth of the lower jaw and the mucosa of the lower oral cavity. Only in this case must the locus of damage be sought laterally in the oral cavity, close to the mandibular angle.

30.1.1 Iatrogenic Damage. The most frequent cause is iatrogenic damage on the occasion of the extraction of the second, and especially of the third, molar tooth. The nerve is damaged by pressure, in which case there is some hope for recovery. Sometimes the nerve is cut during osteotomy or a similar surgical procedure, or during incision of a sublingual abscess or removal of a tumor of the same location.

30.1.2 Circumscribed Neoplastic or Inflammatory Disease of the Posterior Lateral Area of the Oral Cavity. Prior to surgery the inflammatory process might damage the nerve by pressure or toxic activity, and there may be invasion of the nerve by a neighboring tumor.

30.2 Bilateral

30.2.1 Regional Psychogenic Pain. In the case of bilateral numbness or burning pain which is limited to the tongue and does not include alteration in the sense of taste, the most likely diagnosis is regional psychogenic pain. For anatomical reasons it is hard to conceive of a disease process with symmetrical localization in the oral cavity, close to the mandibular angle, and when this bilateral affection does occur, it should lead to a diminished appreciation of taste. These patients need not be overtly depressive; on the contrary, they exhibit emotional responsiveness and undiminished initiative. In all probability they will deny having personal problems. It is useful to confirm the suspected diagnosis by demonstrating attenuation or relief of the symptoms following the administration of thymoleptic or neuroleptic drugs.

30.2.2 Carcinoma of the Upper Throat and Related Disease. One should not, however, rely too heavily on this effect, because even sensory symptoms of *organic origin* are improved by these and other drugs. It is advisable to examine these patients thoroughly by inspection of the upper throat and by neuroimaging of the base of the skull, because more than one of these patients has eventually developed symptoms of the entire mandibular branch of the trigeminal nerve, thus betraying a *malignancy* that had previously gone undetected.

30.2.3 Pernicious Anemia. In rare cases, burning pain of the tongue is the leading symptom of pernicious anemia. The fact that this condition has become quite infrequent might be related to the widespread parenteral application of preparations containing much more than the daily requirement of vitamin B_{12}. These preparations are erroneously believed to give relief from pain of various kinds. So the underlying disease might have been temporarily cured by unwitting substitution for the lack of vitamin B_{12}.

The diagnosis rests on blood tests, including serum level of vitamin B_{12}, examination of absorption of the vitamin in the intestinal tract, and microscopical examination of bone marrow. It should be stressed again that the conditions mentioned in Sects. 30.2.2 and 30.2.3 have to be ruled out before the diagnosis of regional psychogenic pain is made even though statistically this condition is to be expected much more frequently.

31 Sudden Loss of Consciousness

In most cases of sudden loss of consciousness, no recent history is available. Also, remote history which might provide a diagnostic clue is usually rather meager, as persons close to the patient are either too excited or uninformed.

31.1 Syncope

The most common cause is one of the variants of syncope. These are discussed in detail in Chap. 32 in the context of sudden loss of posture. Frequently, not only posture but also consciousness is lost, even though only for a period of seconds. Prolonged unconsciousness is rare.

31.2 Generalized Epileptic Seizure

A postictal state is an apparently simple situation, but the seizure may have gone unnoticed or unreported for various reasons. It is difficult to imagine to what extent the family may be ashamed of their epileptic relative. The typical signs like bitten tongue or lips may be absent. Enuresis may have various causes. A postparoxysmal hemiparesis may mislead the diagnostician if the patient is beyond what is euphemistically called the prime of life (see Chap. 5). Elevation of creatine kinase provides a useful clue.

31.3 Intracerebral Hemorrhage

Intracerebral hemorrhage usually occurs in chronically hypertensive patients. The cause is rupture of a small arteriosclerotic aneurysm; preferred localizations are the basal ganglia, pons, and cerebellum. The patient is found somnolent or unconscious. He is likely to have hemiplegia, which can be assessed in the unconscious patient by unilateral loss of muscle tone. Proprioceptive reflexes may be diminished on the paralyzed side, but Babinski's sign will be present. In hemispheric hemorrhage there is frequently *conjugate deviation of the eyes* toward the side of the brain lesion. In pontine hemorrhage there will be tetraplegia with bilateral extensor reflexes and various oculomotor signs. If there is conjugate deviation of the eyes it is directed away from a unilateral pontine lesion, in contrast to hemispheric damage where it is directed toward the lesion (the hemispheric oculomotor system "pushes" the eyeballs to the contralateral side). "Swimming" conjugate or disconjugate ocular movements are frequent and of little value for localizing lesions within the brain stem. Spontaneous nystagmus is likely to beat horizontally in pontine and vertically in midbrain lesions.

Ocular bobbing is most frequently seen in lower brain stem compression owing to a space-occupying lesion of the cerebellum. It is frequently, but not absolutely certainly, a sign of irreversible brain stem dysfunction. Attenuation of the oculocephalic reflex parallels depth of coma.

Pupillary alterations are frequent. Bilateral miosis indicates damage at the pontine level, if the reaction to light is preserved, and this can sometimes be seen only with a magnifying glass. Unilateral mydriasis is seen when the third nerve nucleus or its autonomic efference in the midbrain tectum are affected. Bilateral mydriasis is an ominous sign. CSF is sanguinolent in most cases. Neuroimaging clearly shows the locus and extent of the hemorrhage and its possible space-occupying effect, which might necessitate neurosurgical intervention.

31.4 Subarachnoid Hemorrhage (SAH)

The diagnosis of SAH is discussed in Chap. 4. Here it is important that some patients are found unconscious after SAH. There is almost always neck stiffness, and lumbar tap will provide hemorrhagic CSF. Centrifugation is standard, because the most experienced doctor may tap a vein, thus causing an artificial admixture of blood to the CSF. Neuroimaging shows SAH, and may even suggest prognosis. Large blood clots give a warning that arterial spasms are to be expected during the next few days. Also, communicating hydrocephalus is recognized early by neuroimaging.

31.5 Basilar Artery Thrombosis

Thrombosis of the basilar artery rarely occurs without premonitory symptoms, which may have been present for several days. Patients are reported to have exhibited slurred speech, diplopia, and ataxia or paresthesia of the limbs. These warning symptoms usually fluctuate until there is sudden or rapidly evolving loss of consciousness. History taking is essential in these cases.

The neurologic findings are similar to those described for pontine hemorrhage. Doppler ultrasound study is most rewarding in these cases, in that lesion of the large vessels leads to an abnormal flow pattern. The most suggestive finding is a high-resistance flow pattern over the vertebral arteries, which is found even in basilar artery occlusion. Transcranial ultrasound examination permits direct measurement of the flow in the basilar artery and is extremely helpful in the evaluation of patients who are candidates for angiography.

Angiography of the hindbrain circulation shows vertebrobasilar stenosis or occlusion, and in particular "top of the basilar artery occlusion", which is of embolic origin.

Acute vertebrobasilar high-grade stenosis or occlusion is susceptible to emergency treatment either by continuous heparin infusion or by intra-arterial thrombolytic therapy.

31.6 Head Trauma

The event may have escaped observation, and the patient is found in coma with any combination of signs described in the preceding paragraphs. It is important to examine any comatose patient for a cranial wound, because in the case of head trauma he is in need of close observation for the development of epidural or subdural hematoma. These complications have to be suspected if coma becomes deeper and hemiplegia evolves.

31.7 Psychogenic

Typical signs of psychogenic "coma" are closure of the eyelids upon the attempt to test oculomotor and pupillomotor functions, conjugate deviation of the bulbs upward upon opening of the closed eyelids, and absence of reaction to painful stimuli in the presence of a preserved blink reflex when the eyelashes are touched. Not all of the possible patterns of behavior can be described here. The important point is that the doctor should develop a feeling for some incongruities in the pattern of the apparently unconscious patient's behavior. The EEG is likely to clarify the situation if one knows how to distinguish the nonreactive EEG in alpha coma from the arousal reaction easily elicited in the waking state.

32 Sudden Loss of Posture
(With and Without Loss of Consciousness)

Rarely does a patient experience sudden loss of posture as an isolated event. Recurrence is the rule, and when the patient is seen by the doctor he is ready to indicate the kind of circumstances that favor the attack, or his relatives are able to do so. Diagnosis rests, to a large extent, on careful history taking.

32.1 Astatic Epileptic Seizures

The onset of astatic epileptic seizures occurs in early infancy, roughly at the age of 2–4 years. The individual attack lasts only a few seconds. The children drop down vertically, do not lose consciousness, and are able to stand up again immediately. The attacks are clustered in series that are separated by free intervals of up to an hour. As a consequence of the great number of attacks, the children bear multiple injuries, and some have their head protected by some kind of thick bandage. Mental development is retarded, and there may be behavioral abnormalities of various kinds. EEG is always pathologic. It shows irregular high-voltage, slow-frequency activity interspersed with sharp waves.

32.2 Common Syncope

The onset of common syncope usually occurs in adolescence or in young adulthood, but the condition may persist long beyond that period. In the initial phase, the situations which trigger it are such that the reason for orthostatic hypotension with failure of the sympathetic, and preponderance of the parasympathetic, innervation of the cardiovascular system is easily recognized. Syncope occurs when the patient jumps to his feet or has to stand relatively immobile for a long time. Emotional strain favors the attacks. Later on, even minor stress is sufficient to trigger the syncope, and psychic influences predominate.

The single attack gradually loses its characteristic features, which are blackout, dizziness, cold sweat, and finally slow sliding to the ground. Rather, the patient falls down abruptly, and during that stage he may lose urine, hurt himself, bite his tongue, and lose consciousness for periods of up to an hour. Under these circumstances it may be difficult to achieve a clinical differentiation from epileptic fits unless one personally observes an attack and finds the patient pale instead of red, the eyes closed instead of open, and the pupils narrow instead of wide, and unreactive. A short tonic stretching of the limbs may occur in syncope, and even some short clonic twitching, thought to be caused by rapidly transient hypoxia of the brain, which causes large populations of nerve cells to fire simultaneously.

EEG is normal as soon as one has the opportunity to record it, and it remains so after sleep deprivation and during long-term recording.

32.3 Cough, Swallowing, and Micturition Syncope

There are some well-defined situations that provoke syncopal attacks. These are coughing, swallowing, or nocturnal micturition all of which favor a fast switch toward a preponderance of parasympathetic tone. Remarkably, these patients do not faint under circumstances other than those in which their syncope is normally triggered. Also, one rarely, if ever, detects psychic influences.

32.4 Carotid Sinus Syndrome

There is relative loss of sympathetic influence both on the heart and on the circulatory system in carotid sinus syndrome, also. The final common mechanism is the same as in syncope, namely, hypoxia of the brain and brain stem, which leads to loss of muscular tone, sometimes fainting, and, rarely, several brief convulsions. The attacks are triggered by turning the head to the side or reclining the head, especially when the patient's collar is too tight, so that pressure is exerted on the carotid sinus. The attacks are seen mostly in persons of advanced age who show signs of atherosclerotic disease.

Diagnosis is verified by compressing the carotid sinus while electrocardiogram and EEG are recorded. It is mandatory that a team is on hand during this maneuvre to reanimate the patient should the test lead to prolonged asystolia. Moreover, CW ultrasound sonography should have demonstrated patency of the carotid artery at the point of pressure, or otherwise there is the risk of releasing an embolus from a local plaque or of provoking acute occlusion of a subtotal carotid stenosis which, in 50% of cases, is accompanied by transport of an embolus into the middle cerebral artery.

32.5 Adams-Stokes Syndrome

In Adams-Stokes syndrome the events described in the preceding three sections are brought about by paroxysmal asystolia lasting longer than 10 s or – very rarely – by paroxysmal tachycardia with a heart rate of more than 180 or 200 per min. In extreme tachycardia the cardiac output is reduced to such an extent that cerebral hypoxia ensues. Diagnosis is provided by the cardiologist. The general practitioner or neurologist should suspect cardiac origin of syncope when the ECG is grossly abnormal.

32.6 Drop Attack

Some authors have described drop attacks as one of the many symptoms of vertebrobasilar insufficiency. Others suggest that the pathophysiology is not very well understood, and they are probably right. Drop attacks occur mainly in middle-aged women.

The patients, who otherwise feel healthy, abruptly drop down and fall on their knees. There is no triggering situation, e.g., abnormal strain on the circulatory system. The patients do not, as a rule, lose consciousness, but are able to get up immediately. They do not experience fainting or abnormality of the heart beat. They describe the attack "as if suddenly the legs no longer have the strength to carry the body." Injury to the knees is frequent.

Ultrasound study of the vertebral circulation rarely reveals gross abnormality, such as a subclavian steal mechanism, or bilateral stenosis of the vertebral artery. All other ancillary examinations are normal.

32.7 Cataplectic Attack

A detailed description of cataplectic attacks is given in Chap. 18. It is sufficient here to mention them as one of the rarer causes of sudden loss of posture.

32.8 Psychogenic Faint

It has already been mentioned above that all too frequently there is gradual transition from syncope resulting from orthostatic malfunction to psychogenic faint. This is not to say that autonomic malfunction has a very strong positive correlation with "psychogenic behavior." One should bear in mind, however, that a personality structure that tends to express itself in "conversion symptoms" may easily find a way to do so if there is a predisposition to a symptom so striking as suddenly falling down. For some patients, not only the young ones, the psychiatrist's skill may be as important as that of the cardiologist.

32.9 Basilar Artery Migraine

In migraine, in particular basilar artery migraine, sudden loss of posture is one of the rare symptoms and, moreover, does not occur during every attack. Usually the patients faint, drop to the floor, and lose consciousness for several seconds. There is nothing alarming in this symptom if it is reported in the context of a history of migraine.

33 Sudden Loss of Speech

If a patient presents with loss of speech of sudden onset, one should try to decide, although this is not of the utmost diagnostic importance, whether he has *anarthria* i.e., loss of the motor faculty to pronounce spoken speech (which requires the coordinated activities of respiration, phonation, and articulation), or whether he is *aphasic*, i.e., has a supramodal disturbance of language.

This is not an easy task even when the patient is alert and cooperative, which is rarely the case in any acute illness. Simple questions are likely to elicit Yes/No answers, thus bringing about a 50% chance of guessing. Furthermore, even aphasic patients are remarkably good in grasping the meaning of the partner's utterance by applying a key word strategy, helped by their situational ("pragmatic") knowledge and understanding, which is not impaired by the linguistic disturbance.

Examination with simple commands will be hindered if the patient is hemiplegic and/or bedridden. In addition, concomitant apraxia may be a limiting factor. Even apparently simple commands like "open your mouth" or "stick out your tongue" can not be obeyed by a patient with oral apraxia.

Reading is hard to test, because it requires a spoken gestural or motor reaction, but writing might help toward the right decision. If the patient has right-sided hemiplegia a very useful test is to provide him with rectangular sheets of paper bearing the constituents of a sentence, which he has to place in the correct order. Even the experienced aphasiologist, however, will have to postpone his decision in some instances, e.g., when the patient does not even attempt to utter a sound. The doctor must, however, be aware, that as time goes by the picture might change and an aphasia present at the day of admission might clear rapidly and give way to dysarthria, i.e., a purely motor disorder of speech. For the neurologic diagnosis, much depends on the patient's age.

33.1 Complicated Migraine

In a young person we suspect in the first place an attack of complicated migraine. The typical combination of signs and symptoms is the following: acute or subacute loss of speech, more often than not without hemiplegia, followed by headache which the patient has experienced periodically before and which may or may not have been accompanied by neurologic signs. If this is his first migrainous attack, the family history is helpful when available, because the condition is familial in 60% of cases.

The EEG is likely to show circumscribed slow waves in the left temporoparietal area, which may persist for as long as 3 weeks, while neuroimaging remains normal. Severe focal EEG alterations in the presence of normal neuroimaging on the 2nd day are virtually diagnostic, except in cases of herpes simplex encephalitis (see below). It must be understood that there should be no cardiac bruits suggestive of cerebral embolism, which might occur in all age groups. A possible source of embolism will be confirmed or ruled out by ultrasound cardiac examination. Vascular bruits on the neck are rather unreliable, as compared with Doppler ultrasound sonography. Transcranial Doppler ultrasound sonography should be applied if available. If the migrainous patient is in the 40- to 50-year-old age group an asymptomatic stenosing vascular lesion might be present but the typical headache, the rapid amelioration of signs and symptoms, and the absence of structural changes in neuroimaging study in contrast to the EEG alterations described above will permit the correct diagnosis. Examination of CSF is not necessary unless the signs and symptoms are progressive.

33.2 Left Hemispheric Stroke

In the elderly, stroke is the most likely diagnosis. In most instances of loss of speech due to stroke, there will be right-sided hemiparesis or hemiplegia, hemisensory impairment and sometimes even hemianopia, or at least right-sided visual neglect. In these cases all the diagnostic considerations and procedures described in Chap. 5 come into play, in particular neuroimaging, which is the only way to reliably distinguish between intracranial hemorrhage and ischemic stroke.

Loss of speech is almost always due to left hemispheric stroke. It might occur also in right (i.e., non-language-dominant) hemispheric stroke, but in this case will clear much faster, and recovery will probably be complete.

Basilar artery insufficiency might severely impair speech articulation, but will render the patient mute only in the case of basilar artery occlusion leading to akinetic mutism, which is a rather rare event.

In the first stages of vertebrobasilar insufficiency, the impairment in spoken speech is characterized mainly by disturbances in respiration and vocalization and the effects of flaccid paralysis of the articulators. With some experience it is easy to distinguish between "bulbar" and "hemispheric" dysarthria.

33.3 Postictal State

In all age groups beyond infancy, loss of speech may be a postictal phenomenon. The epileptic fit may have gone unrecognized, even without biting of the tongue or lips, and increased blood level of creatine kinase is indicative if present, but is not a reliable finding.

The EEG quite often provides a diagnostic clue (slow and sharp waves, generalized or focal). The loss of speech will quickly resolve and leave the diagnostician with the task of finding out why the patient has had an epileptic seizure (see Chap. 14).

33.4 Brain Tumor or Abscess

The history of patients harboring a brain tumor or abscess may be completely unrevealing: no headache, no loss of initiative or flattening of affect, and no easily detectable inflammatory ENT (ear, nose, and throat) process. Sudden loss of speech is brought about by rupture of a feeding vessel and hemorrhage into the tumor, by rapid increase of perifocal edema, or, in the case of left hemispheric tumor or abscess, by a partial or generalized epileptic seizure. Only systematic investigation of the patient will lead to the correct diagnosis. EEG is a necessary measure, with the following possible findings:

- Localized slowing, which is ambiguous. However, very slow waves in the subdelta range, accompanied by general slowing of electrical activity, are suggestive of brain abscess.
- Local slow waves in the delta or theta range may be indicative of a hemispheric tumor.

CT scan will show a space-occupying lesion of low density with or without a ring formation (uptake of contrast), both in brain tumor and brain abscess. Abscesses are likely to produce more widespread edema.

33.5 Thrombosis of Intracerebral Sinus

The typical triad suggesting sinus thrombosis is partial or generalized epileptic fits, focal hemispheric signs, and decrease in vigilance. EEG shows widespread slow activity of low amplitude over an entire hemisphere with distribution also over the other hemisphere. In neuroimaging, sinus thrombosis is recognizable by hemispheric swelling with predominantly parasagittal localization, diapedesis bleeding, primary hyperdensity of the sinus(es), and delta-shaped sparing of the confluens sinuum after the injection of contrast.

33.6 Herpes Simplex Encephalitis

The clinical picture of HSV encephalitis is described in Chap. 14. Since the temporal lobe is primarily affected, aphasia is a frequent initial sign. EEG shows focal slowing, which evolves on repeated recording to periodic triphasic complexes. These eventually show also over the frontal and contralateral leads. Neuroimaging shows an area of low density, which soon acquires space-occupying characteristics and spreads from deep temporal to frontal areas and eventually to the contralateral side, affecting in the first place areas belonging to the limbic system. CSF shows "inflammatory signs." Unfortunately, demonstration of HSV infection, either by direct visualization of virus particles or by ELISA technique, provides positive findings only with considerable delay, with the result that virostatic therapy has to be initiated as soon as there is a strong suspicion of the diagnosis. After all, lethality is as high as 85% in HSV encephalitis, so this is a case for a calculated risk.

34 Symmetrical Areflexia

The presence or absence of proprioceptive reflexes per se has no functional significance. Chronic absence of the ankle jerk after recovery from a slipped disk does not make the gait awkward, nor does it impair rapid alternating movements of the feet. Nevertheless, symmetrical lack of reflexes indicates that there is or has been an affection of the peripheral nervous system, and therefore calls for a thorough neurologic and medical examination. Symmetrical attenuation of reflexes in the lower limbs relative to the upper limbs and to the masseter jerk, the only clinically relevant proprioceptive reflex in the distribution of the cranial nerves, has to be treated along the same lines.

34.1 Polyneuropathy

The most frequent cause is polyneuropathy. All the variants that have an acute onset will hardly escape diagnostic attention, because there is weakness and/or sensory disturbance of the affected limbs or the trunk. So the problem does not lie in determining whether the patient has polyneuropathy, but rather in recognizing its etiology.

34.1.1 Guillain-Barré Syndrome. There are clear-cut criteria for the diagnosis of Guillain-Barré syndrome, the most important of which are acute or subacute onset (the rare chronic variant will be discussed below); predominance of motor over sensory signs and symptoms; ascending distribution with eventual inclusion of the proximal (girdle), abdominal, truncal, and respiratory muscles; frequent occurrence of bilateral facial palsy; slowing of nerve conduction; and the CSF finding of an increase in the protein level in the presence of a normal cell count. The possible complications are discussed in Chaps. 20 and 23.

A medical and, in particular, serological examination for a recognizable cause is mandatory, the most frequent causes being Epstein-Barr virus infection, epidemic hepatitis type B, or immunopathy, or an other hematological disease. The latter conditions have to be taken into account when the pattern of signs and symptoms is atypical, e.g., very pronounced sensory symptoms, descending course, or increase in CSF cell count. Among the rare causes of acute polyneuropathy listed are alcoholism with severe malnutrition and vitamin B_1 deficiency, and polyarteritis, both of which usually lead to chronic polyneuropathy.

34.1.2 Chronic Polyneuropathy. It is possible for chronic polyneuropathy to go undetected for a long time, because the patient does not have characteristic complaints or does not take his symptoms seriously, and the signs have to be looked for by neurologic examination.

Many patients with *diabetes mellitus* have diminished or absent ankle jerks and/or patellar reflexes, their calf and pretibial muscles are slightly atrophic, and the extensor digitorum brevis muscle on the dorsolateral aspect of the foot directly in front of the lateral ankle may not be palpable when the patient performs an extensor (dorsal) movement of the toes. Frequently, the patient does not feel the vibration of the tuning fork on his big toe or ankle. Nerve conduction study will reveal generalized slowing of motor and sensory conduction, suggesting a disorder in the metabolism of the myelin sheaths.

It is true that this "subclinical affection of the peripheral nervous system does not immediately threaten the patient's health. However, it clearly indicates that the metabolic derangement is not adequately controlled, be it on the dietary or on the medical side, or in both respects. Some authors submit that a diabetic patient who develops polyneuropathy under strict diet and adequate oral therapy is a case for treatment with insulin.

The recognition of subclinical polyneuropathy in confused or delirious patients may help the identification of *alcoholism* as the cause of the psychiatric disorder. Chronic alcohol abuse leads to polyneuropathy characterized clinically by attenuation of proprioceptive reflexes and mild paresis of lower limb muscles, in particular of the extensors (see Chaps. 15 and 16), without striking sensory symptoms. Electrophysiological studies show axonal damage recognizable by denervation potentials in needle myography in the presence of normal or near-normal nerve conduction velocity.

Complete medical examination of a patient whose subclinical chronic polyneuropathy does not fall into one of the above-mentioned categories, where the incidence is relatively high, is time-consuming, costly, and frequently frustrating. The following list includes some of the rarer etiologies:

– Renal failure
– Paraneoplastic, rheumatoid, or lupoid arteritis

- Porphyria
- Vitamin deficiency (B_1, B_6, B_{12})
- Exogenous intoxication, e.g., by lead, thallium, or arsenic

34.2 Combined Degeneration of the Spinal Cord

Vitamin B_{12} deficiency is an important cause of areflexia, because it is a treatable condition. The diagnosis is strongly suggested if the patient presents with the full-blown picture of combined degeneration of the spinal cord, i.e., weakness, areflexia, and stocking-and-glove distribution of sensory symptoms in the presence of plantar extensor responses, indicating affection of the pyramidal tracts (see Chap. 29).

34.3 Charcot-Marie-Tooth Disease
(Hereditary Motor Sensory Neuropathy Type I)

Not in every case does attenuation or absence of reflexes indicate polyneuropathy. There are inborn degenerative diseases which are summarized today under the name of hereditary motor sensory neuropathy (HMSN). The variant that was formerly described as Charcot-Marie-Tooth disease may take a very mild course and appear as a "forme fruste", where there is only areflexia and perhaps some reversible deformity of the foot (hollow foot). The diagnosis is easy if one considers the contrast between the sriking signs (absence of reflexes, drastic reduction in nerve conduction velocity) and the almost total lack of complaint by the patient, as well as the lack of denervation in needle EMG. It is most valuable to examine close relatives of the patient, who, as a rule, show the same pattern as he does.

34.4 Spinocerebellar Ataxia (Atrophy)

Similar considerations apply to the variants of spinocerebellar ataxia (atrophy), another group of hereditary degenerative diseases. The traditional distinction between a juvenile and primarily spinal form, frequently named Friedreich's ataxia, and an adult, primarily cerebellar, variant named after Nonne and Pierre Marie certainly simplifies the real situation. There are more intermediate than classical cases. The leading syndrome is locomotor ataxia of insidious onset and slow but relentless course toward deterioration. Reflexes are frequently absent. Family history may be unremarkable. Neuroimaging findings are unreliable. One must not expect to find cerebellar atrophy even when there is striking cerebellar ataxia.

34.5 Adie's Syndrome

If the pupils are strongly asymmetrical and the larger one appears to react neither to light nor to convergence/near sight, one should consider the possibility that this is a case of *tonic pupil*, and, if there is areflexia, that the patient may have Adie's syndrome. Sometimes the patient has noticed the pupillary abnormality himself. He may have felt increased sensibility to the brightness of the sun, which is due to lack of pupillary contraction in reaction to the light stimulus, or he may have had blurred vision when attempting to read, which is due to absence of immediate accommodation. Some patients notice one morning when looking in the mirror that "one eye looks different."

The asymmetry and lack of response of the pupil suggests to the doctor the diagnosis of neurosyphilis, because areflexia is present. However, serological reactions are negative, and ophthalmologic examination demonstrates preserved but very slow reaction of the pupil. The cause of the condition is degeneration of the parasympathetic cells in the ciliary ganglion. Because there is parasympathetic denervation of the pupil there is also, of course, denervation hypersensitivity to cholinergic agents. This can easily be demonstrated by prompt narrowing of the affected pupil upon the application of a weak solution of a cholinergic agent, while the normal, not hypersensitive pupil does not contract (see Chap. 29).

34.6 Tabes Dorsalis

Sometimes areflexia is found in a patient who presents with pupillary abnormalities. If both pupils are miotic, slightly eccentric, and do not react to light but do react on convergence and show accommodation to near sight, this is in all likelihood a case of tabes dorsalis. It is then necessary to establish by lumbar tap and serological examination of serum and CSF whether the syphilitic affection is still active, in which case it requires penicillin treatment, or whether the disease has burnt itself out and there is no need for treatment. The same considerations apply if the pupils are large, slightly unequal, and show the same pattern of reaction as described above.

34.7 Motor Neuron Disease

In rare instances, motor neuron disease presents with areflexia of the legs. The diagnosis is made according to the following criteria: only motor, and no sensory, signs and symptoms, fasciculation in affected, i.e., weak, muscles, and frequently also in nonaffected muscles, and generalized denervation in EMG study in contrast to normal or near-normal nerve conduction velocity. Since this is a very grave diagnosis, motor neuron disease being an incurable, relentlessly progressing disease, it is advisable to do two things:

1. Perform biopsy of a mildly affected muscle and of the purely sensory sural nerve, unless the diagnosis is established beyond doubt, e.g., by the presence of bulbar paralysis with fasciculation of the tongue and disturbance of articulation, phonation, and respiration, while the masseter jerk is brisk. The rationale for biopsy is that motor neuron disease does not affect sensory nerves, so neuropathological examination should yield a normal result.
2. Examine the patient carefully for syphilis or a malignancy, with a view to establishing secondary motor neuron disease.

35 Transverse Syndrome of the Spinal Cord

More often than not, the transverse syndrome of the spinal cord is incomplete; in other words, some motor, sensory, and/or autonomic functions below the presumed level of damage are preserved. If this holds true for all sensory or motor modalities, no conclusion as to the localization and nature of the underlying disease process can be drawn on clinical grounds alone. There is one characteristic syndrome, however, that strongly suggests a lesion at the ventral aspect of the cord, namely, the so-called *anterior spinal artery syndrome.*

The anterior spinal artery, which travels longitudinally along the ventral surface of the cord, supplies the anterior two-thirds of the cord via a great number of sulcocommissural arteries that enter the cord in roughly ventrodorsal direction. These irrigate the anterior and lateral horns, and the spinothalamic, anterior, and, more importantly, lateral corticospinal tracts. The crucial point is that the posterior columns are not affected. Consequently, the anterior spinal artery syndrome (which is identical with the syndrome of a central lesion within the spinal cord) consists of the following signs and symptoms:

- Central paraparesis of the lower limbs, which may be flaccid in the acute phase, but eventually exhibits spastic increase of muscle tone
- Inability to empty the bladder, which eventually evolves into an overflow bladder
- Decreased awareness of painful stimuli and inability to appreciate the temperature of external stimuli

In contrast, touch may be felt and correctly localized, and the vibration of a tuning fork is appreciated. The syndrome is unspecific, but it provides diagnostic clues, the elaboration of which is discussed in the first two sections of this chapter.

35.1 Occlusion of the Anterior Spinal Artery

The artery may be occluded by an embolus or by local atherosclerotic disease. Onset of signs and symptoms is acute. The incomplete transverse lesion of the spinal cord occurs at lower cervical or thoracic levels where large feeding vessels join the anterior spinal artery. Most patients are of advanced age and show signs of generalized atherosclerosis. CSF and x-ray examinations are normal. Sometimes there is elevation of hematocrit, as in cerebral stroke.

35.2 Vertebral Disease

Compression of the cord may be the consequence of vertebral disease that leads to the destruction of the affected vertebra and the intrusion of osseous, neoplastic, or inflammatory tissue into the spinal canal. History may or may not reveal that the patient had experienced radicular ("girdle") pain at the level of damage some time prior to the acute event. Quite frequently, however, the partial transverse syndrome develops with no warning. Neurologic examination can only roughly reveal the locus of lesion. It is more reliable as an indicator of the transverse localization than of the level of damage. The reason is the so-called eccentric arrangement of long ascending and descending fiber tracts. Any lesion affecting the cord from its peripheral toward its central portions is likely to interfere first with those long fiber tracts, with the result that the clinical localization is usually lower than the actual damage.

Some of the laboratory findings, such as sedimentation rate, are of immediate value. Others, such as indicators of osseous metabolism, are not available on the spot.

Consequently, only ancillary examinations help to assess the diagnosis. X-ray of the vertebral column and neuroimaging in conventional and in bone window study will reveal destruction of vertebrae due to neoplastic or inflammatory disease. Isotope scan of the vertebral column is of help, should x-ray and neuroimaging be unremarkable. Isotope studies are useful as searching methods when the level of damage to the column cannot otherwise be identified. If the level is recognized, myelography in combination with CT scan will demonstrate the extent of medullary compression and, possibly, extraspinal tumor invasion.

35.3 Extramedullary Tumor

Myelography combined with CT scan is very useful in the identification of extramedullary, intradural space-occupying lesions. The vertebral column is patent in these cases, yet there is compression of the spinal cord. Myelography has the advantage of providing a good visualization of the location of the disease process, together with CSF findings that may be most revealing. The spectrum of disease processes ranges from neurinoma or meningioma (usually located on the laterodorsal aspect of the cord and requiring neurosurgical intervention) to lymphoma, which is quite susceptible to x-ray treatment.

35.4 Herniated Disc

A herniated cervical disc usually leads to Brown-Séquard's syndrome (see Chap. 8), but it may also produce an anterior spinal cord syndrome. There need not be a "typical releasing event"; the majority of cases I have seen occurred in most unremarkable situations, sometimes while the patient was stretching out the arms in a supine position. Neuroimaging is the first choice among the ancillary methods.

35.5 Myelitis

A more or less complete, at any rate unsystematic, lesion of the spinal cord is brought about by inflammatory disease of the cord itself. Myelitis may be of viral etiology; in other words, it occurs as a postinfectious immune reaction presenting as multilocular perivenous demyelination. This condition is not easily differentiated from multiple sclerosis if the criteria listed in Chap. 10 are not met. Given that postinfectious myelitis usually takes a benign course and does not recur, and given, furthermore, that the early diagnosis of multiple sclerosis has no medical and frequently only slight social consequences, it may not appear to be a matter of great urgency to establish the diagnosis one way or the other.

35.6 Epidural Hemorrhage

An acute transverse syndrome of the spinal cord in a patient receiving cumarin is most probably due to epidural hemorrhage. These patients should immediately be given drugs antagonizing the effect of cumarin, because they require neuroimaging, myelography, and immediate operation.

35.7 Epidural Abscess

This disease is characterized by an incomplete transverse syndrome of progressive nature: localized pain that is almost intolerable, accompanied by a stiffness of the affected part of the vertebral column;

local tenderness; and "inflammatory alterations" of the blood tests. There is no time for any ancillary examinations except x-ray and myelography. Neurosurgical treatment is urgent.

35.8 Spinal Angioma

The diagnosis of spinal angioma is quite complex. Textbooks suggest that signs and symptoms fluctuate for a long period of time. In reality, history is often quite uncharacteristic, and there is only an indication of progressive spinal cord damage that is not clearly localized. These patients have bladder disturbances. The fact that there is progressive illness with spinal cord pathology of no precise localization will prompt myelography, particularly as there are no signs permitting the exact localization necessary for a reasonable neuroimaging examination. If myelography suggests the presence of a vascular malformation, spinal angiography is required.

35.9 Late Traumatic Compression of the Spinal Cord

An acute traumatic lesion of the spinal cord is easily recognizable from the patient's history. Chronic vascular myelopathy following compression fracture of a vertebra may be difficult to diagnose without x-ray, because the patient will not suspect a trauma he suffered years ago to be the cause of the progressive spinal cord syndrome, and may therefore forget to report it.

35.10 Intramedullary Tumor of the Spinal Cord

Intrinsic tumors of the spinal cord are rare. Paresthesias, paraparesis, and micturition disturbances are more prominent than pain. Consequently, a spinal variant of multiple sclerosis is suspected, if neurologic disease is considered at all. There is, however, neither multiplicity in time nor in space. The progressive course of spinal disease affecting multiple systems (sensory, motor, autonomic) should prompt the search for a space-occupying lesion.

36 Tremor at Rest

Tremor at rest occurs first in the most distal parts of the limbs. Frequently, it can be observed in the toes and in the fingers, and this has great diagnostic significance if one has to differentiate between organic and psychogenic tremor. The latter is not very likely to manifest itself in the lower extremities, because these have no expressive function as long as the patient is not walking about.

36.1 Parkinson's Disease

Parkinsonian tremor has an alternating beat in antagonistic muscles, with a frequency of 4–6/s. The most common form is rhythmic flexion and extension of the semiflexed fingers, which eventually spreads proximally to result in flexor/extensor movements at the wrist. Only in very advanced stages does the tremor affect the muscles acting on the elbow joint, and it is rarely, if ever, seen in shoulder movements. The same applies to the toes and feet. The tremor may start in one limb only and may be confined to it or become more pronounced after later bilateral involvement over a long period of time.

The tremor diminishes greatly or stops completely upon voluntary movement of the affected limb, but reappears after termination of that movement. This is probably due to a desynchronizing effect of the pyramidal tract on the anterior horn cells.

There is no problem in recognizing parkinsonian tremor as such if the patient has one or all of the other characteristic features of Parkinson's syndrome: cogwheel rigidity, which betrays a disturbance in reciprocal innervation (and relaxation) of muscles; and akinesia with paucity of expressive, associated, and, in an advanced stage, also of voluntary movements, to name but the prominent ones. If, however, tremor is the only obvious sign, differential diagnosis is dfficult, and

139

sometimes one has to observe the further course of the condition before reaching a decision. Characteristic traits of parkinsonian tremor are: stable frequency of 4–6/s; machinelike action at rest; attenuation on voluntary movement which is seen even prior to the execution of a planned purposeful movement; and increase in amplitude, but not in frequency, during emotional tension. When the affected limb is passively held firm by the examiner, tremor may start in another limb.

36.2 Benign, Essential, or Familial Tremor

The onset of benign, essential, or familial tremor usually occurs during the first 2 decades of life, i.e., much earlier than any variant of Parkinson's syndrome, except Wilson's disease (see below). There is alternating tremor at rest, the frequency of which is only slightly faster than in parkinsonism (5–9/s). It is likewise increased by emotion, but also, in contrast to parkinsonism, during voluntary movement. Usually, it does not start in one hand only, and there is frequently also a fine resting tremor of the head. Familial tremor is attenuated by alcohol intake, but this may also be true in other types of tremor.

The most characteristic feature is that over the years the tremor may become coarser, but there will be no rigidity, akinesia, or any other sign of "extrapyramidal" disease. In most cases the diagnosis may be supported *ex juvantibus*, because beta-receptor blocking agents will improve the tremor dramatically.

36.3 Toxic Tremor

Various toxic agents produce a fine tremor which is most clearly seen in the outstretched hands, although it may already be present at rest. The tremor is seen in the distal musculature of the limbs. It is irregular in both frequency and amplitude, and does not diminish during voluntary action.

36.3.1 Alcohol Abuse. The most frequent cause is alcohol abuse. In the first stage it is present only in the morning, and ceases toward evening. This tremor is a withdrawal phenomenon, which is due to nocturnal interruption of regular alcohol intake. It is diagnostic to have the patient confirm this variability, because very few alcoholics are willing to admit to their abuse. In an advanced stage tremor has become permanent and will even be present after a long interruption in alcohol intake. These patients are usually conspicuous by their physical signs, e.g., ectatic veins, scleral jaundice, palpable liver, and a particularly accommodating attitude.

36.3.2 Neuroleptic and Thymoleptic Drugs. Chronic intake of neuroleptic and even more so of thymoleptic drugs produces a similar tremor which, however, owing to the longer half-life of the drugs, does not show striking circadian variations. An exhaustive list would also have to include sedatives of various sorts. Tremor is a characteristic side effect of lithium preparations, which are prescribed to prevent bouts of manic-depressive illness. In an advanced stage of abuse, tremor owing to drugs may be accompanied by slurred speech, which is not a feature of chronic alcohol abuse.

36.3.3 Heavy Metal Intoxication. Among other organs, the brain is affected by heavy metal intoxication, which leads to a fine, fast, irregular tremor. Usually the patients are pale, blood tests show hypochromic anemia, and, in the case of lead intoxication, basophilic inclusions in the erythrocytes.

36.3.4 Thyrotoxic Tremor. Thyrotoxic tremor beats fine and fast, is limited to the most distal parts of the limbs, and is accompanied by other signs of increased sympathetic activity, such as tachycardia, increased sweating, and weight loss.

36.4 Senile Tremor

"Senile tremor" is a term loosely used for tremor in elderly persons who do not necessarily show signs and symptoms of parkinsonism, or of vascular disease of the brain, nor do they report cerebrovascular accidents. There need not be arterial hypertension, and frequently these persons do not even exhibit striking forgetfulness or emotional lability. While the pathophysiology of senile tremor remains unclear, its appearance is rather characteristic. It is a relatively coarse irregular tremor at rest, which ceases when the affected muscles become completely relaxed and increases when a certain position is assumed and a movement performed. Thus, the tremor has features of resting, postural, and action tremor. The condition is socially embarrassing, but from the medical point of view, benign.

36.5 Wilson's Disease

A disturbance in copper metabolism, Wilson's disease is a multifaceted condition that invariably affects the basal ganglia and brain stem, where deposits of copper interfere with normal neural function. In some patients the syndrome resembles multiple sclerosis, in some there is flapping tremor, and in others there is juvenile parkinsonism with resting tremor and akinesia. Wilson's disease must be considered in every patient below the age of 40 who presents with resting tremor. The diagnosis is made on the basis of deposits of copper in the cornea, which are seen under the slit lamp as the greenish Kayser-Fleisher ring, and by demonstration of a diminished serum level of ceruloplasmin and increased urin excretion of copper and various amino acids (see also Chap. 11).

36.6 Psychogenic Tremor

Not infrequently, tremor has a psychic origin. The diagnosis of psychogenic tremor is rather difficult to verify, even though the suspicion may arise early in the diagnostic procedure. There are many pitfalls in the attempt to judge the personality of a patient who presents with an unusual disorder, motor or otherwise. The tremor has elements of most of the varieties so far discussed. It is present at rest and is usually irregular in frequency and amplitude; it increases when the patient assumes a posture, aims at a target, and holds an object. It is not accompanied by other signs of basal ganglia (rigidity, akinesia) or cerebellar disease (nystagmus, dysarthria). Writing movements are usually grossly altered, to such a degree that script becomes all but illegible. There is no micrographia as in Parkinson's disease, or "regular irregularity" as in cerebellar disease, but the lines show abrupt excursions if the patient manages to write at all.

Biofeedback procedures may considerably improve the tremor, much more than is possible in tremor of organic origin.

37 Twilight State

The term "twilight state" denotes a psychopathologic alteration characterized by reduced vigilance and, consequently, reactivity, frequently accompanied by disorientation in time and space. The patients give the overall impression of being slow in mentation and of acting hesitantly, and they obviously do not fully assess their actual social situation. The conditions discussed in this chapter do not all have the same status with regard to the single components of the syndrome. Yet they should be considered if a patient becomes conspicuous mainly by the psychopathological signs and symptoms indicated above.

37.1 Petit Mal Status

An uninterrupted series of simple partial seizures of the absence type, petit mal status is seen mainly in infants and young adults, but may occur in any age group if the patient has had petit mal epilepsy before. Usually, the patients appear not to be fully awake. They have to be addressed repeatedly, and their answers, like their spontaneous actions, are hesitant, often inappropriate, and sometimes perseveratory. On close inspection one might notice rhythmic, clonic closure of the eyes, rhythmic elevation of the ocular bulbs, and sometimes also rhythmic twitching of the upper limbs. These motor phenomena greatly facilitate the diagnosis, which is confirmed by EEG showing continuous 3-cps spike and wave activity over all leads. Intravenous injection of clonazepam quickly resolves the condition, and this effect is diagnostic.

37.2 Complex Partial Seizure Status

Likewise, complex partial seizures may follow each other in an uninterrupted succession. Unfortunately, the clinical picture is much less uniform and does not necessarily include the well-known automatic oral movements and stereotypic actions of the single seizure. Diagnosis relies very much on the EEG, which is highly suggestive of temporal lobe epilepsy. Again, intravenous treatment, in this case preferably with phenytoin, brings the twilight state to an end.

37.3 Postconvulsive Twilight State

Sometimes a grand mal seizure is not noticed, and the patient is found with clouded consciousness, with disorientation, rather tense, and prone to aggressive (re)actions, which have their origin in a profound misunderstanding of the social situation. As described in Chap. 14 the routine signs of an epileptic seizure – bitten tongue, enuresis, and elevation of creatine kinase – may be lacking. Again, EEG will show generalized dysrhythmic slow activity with occasional sharp waves or other elements frequently seen in epileptic disease. Owing to his tension and mistrust, however, it might be impossible to persuade the patient to tolerate the examination. If possible, intravenous injection of clonazepam or phenytoin should be given. In contrast to epileptic disease, the other conditions listed in the table will be much less, if at all, attenuated by these drugs.

37.4 Post-traumatic Twilight State

The diagnosis of post-traumatic twilight state is easy when the patient has sustained a severe head injury with prolonged coma. Upon regaining consciousness the patient may become agitated and often anxious, is disoriented, can not assess his situation, and is given to misinterpretation of surrounding objects. The support for intravenous infusion becomes a threatening figure, and any voice outside the patient's room is interpreted as a summons or a threat. The patient is likely to leave the bed and also the ward, even if suffering from a broken leg. Only a very inexperienced person will judge this behavior as improper conduct.

There are rare instances, however, where a twilight state does not occur after, but in place of, post-traumatic coma. Immediately after trauma, the patient does not seem to realize the situation, and does not know what has happened, or how he came to be at that place. He will not follow the suggestions of others, but is inclined to leave, and walk or drive about aimlessly. Eventually the patient will reach his home and fall asleep there. On waking up, he has retrograde amnesia.

37.5 Poriomania

When the trauma has occurred in a traffic accident caused by the patient, the differential diagnosis has to exclude psychogenic poriomania. The doctor who sees the patient after the condition has cleared has little chance of arriving at a reliable conclusion. One important clue is a pathologic EEG recording on the first examination, and the demonstration of a return to normal on follow-up.

Poriomania is seen more frequently without preceding trauma, and these patients may travel to distant places by car, train, or plane without arousing any suspicion. Days after their departure, they suddenly "wake up" and declare they do not know where they are or how they got there. The majority of reported cases have turned out to be psychogenic. I have seen one patient, though, who traveled 800 km by train in petit mal status and eventually became conspicuous by helpless behavior when the train stopped at a station. The diagnosis was confirmed by EEG.

37.6 Transient Global Amnesia

Sudden onset of helpless behavior is a characteristic feature of transient global amnesia. The condition starts abruptly, mostly without any recognizable cause. Patients no longer recognize their surroundings; they do not remember ongoing events, with the result that time and again they ask the same questions; and they repeatedly forget what they were asked to do and the answers that were given to them. They are disoriented with regard to time and often also to place, and they have retrograde amnesia of varying length. In contrast to these psychological alterations, patients may perform routine activities quite normally. As a rule, physical examination is unremarkable.

Over a period of up to two days, they return to normal again, although they remain amnesic in respect of the episode and sometimes there is retrograde amnesia for a short period prior to the event.

37.7 Encephalitis

Encephalitis is a disease that imitates many conditions, as may be seen with the help of the index to this book. Signs and symptoms may consist only of slight attenuation of wakefulness, flattening of affect, disorientation, and slowing of mentation. In most cases EEG shows generalized alteration – usually slow activity with high-voltage theta waves. Neuroimaging is normal, at least in the initial stage, and CSF contains slight, if any, pleocytosis, and elevation of protein, normal glucose, and low lactate levels (see also Chap. 14).

37.8 Exogenous Psychosis

Finally, any psychotic state owing to metabolic derangement or intoxication has to be considered. The reader is referred to Chap. 3. The most frequent cause in elderly patients is dehydration during an infectious disease, or following an operation. The hematocrit level is elevated. The twilight state usually clears after intravenous administration of saline and glucose solutions. In some patients with small-vessel disease of the brain, general anesthesia produces confusion or a twilight state.

38 Unilateral Fits Affecting Limb(s) or Face

38.1 Jacksonian Fits and Other Partial Motor Seizures

Faced with a complaint of unilateral fit(s) the first task is to establish whether the patient has had similar events before. The next is to find out whether the seizure(s) was (were) motor or sensory, or both. Motor seizures may be tonic or clonic, or may consist of a brief tonic phase which is followed by clonic twitchings. It is useful to learn whether or not there was a *jacksonian march*, which is a slow progression of clonic twitching or paresthesia, usually from proximal to distal parts of the limb. If the arm is affected, the motor or sensory phenomena may spread to the face or to the ipsilateral leg, while the trunk is usually spared. Many patients can clearly describe the progressive march of the jerks or the paresthesia, but very few can describe how the fit ends after a few minutes. There may or may not be Todd's paralysis, i.e., weakness and clumsiness of the affected limb(s) for a period of up to half an hour. Todd's paralysis can also follow a purely sensory jacksonian march. When the seizure and the postictal paresis are over, the patient frequently has only minimal symptoms or neurologic signs, or none at all, which is why he will not see the doctor after the first fit, but rather dismiss it as a trivial event.

The differential diagnosis of jacksonian fits includes principally space-occupying lesions of all varieties, arteriovenous malformations, and thrombosis of the cerebral sinus(es). Examination by neuroimaging with and without contrast is therefore indispensable, followed, if necessary, by cerebral angiography. Of course, any circumscribed lesion affecting the pre- or postcentral gyrus or their neighboring areas may give rise to jacksonian fits, e.g., traumatic brain damage.

An interesting possibility is complicated migraine, which can imitate sensory jacksonian fits. Migraine should be suspected when the symptoms are purely sensory; when they last longer than 10 min (sometimes even hours); and when they are followed by throbbing headache. Most suggestive is the occurrence in young adulthood and in the context of a personal and family history of migraine, and alternation of the affected side of the body. These patients typically have circumscribed slow waves in the EEG, while neuroimaging is normal.

Except for migraine, the above-mentioned considerations hold true also for other variants of partial motor seizures.

38.2 Epilepsia Partialis Continua

Continuous twitching in single muscles or in very circumscribed groups of muscles, such as the triangular or obicularis oculi muscles in the face or the flexor muscles of the thumb, which continues for hours or even days in the fully conscious patient, is called *Koshevnikoff's epilepsy*, or epilepsia partialis continua. It is caused by either structural alteration or metabolic derangement of the brain. A small space-occupying lesion, most probably metastatic or carcinomatous meningitis, should be suspected first. Encephalitis is a much rarer cause. Among the metabolic disorders, one should look for derangement of glucose metabolism. Remarkably enough, common causes are both hypoglycemia and the nonketotic hyperosmolar diabetic condition which need not necessarily lead to coma.

38.3 Stroke

Not only may stroke be heralded by partial seizures, but a sensory stroke beginning with fluctuating symptoms may even somewhat resemble a series of partial seizures. If the duration of sensory symptoms is of the order of transient ischemic attacks, clinical differentiation may be next to impossible, especially since Todd's paralysis cannot be distinguished from the weakness of incipient stroke. Lack of response to intravenously administered clonazepam is of diagnostic significance and strongly speaks against partial seizures. However, the condition of these patients urgently calls for ancillary examinations, mainly EEG, CW ultrasound sonography, and neuroimaging.

38.4 Paroxysmal Kinesigenic Choreoathetosis

Seizures induced by movement, or paroxysmal kinesigenic choreoathetosis, should be discussed in this context. These involuntary movements affect one arm or both ipsilateral extremities without alteration of consciousness (i.e., with preserved wakefulness). They are not tonic-clonic but rather choreoathetotic, i.e., they are slow, mostly extensor, often tortuous, and inimitable movements, which are produced by attempts to move the extremities in deliberate actions. The onset of signs and symptoms usually occurs in childhood, and frequently there is a positive family history. The seizures may recur as often as hundred times a day. EEG is normal during the seizure. Yet, as a rule, there is a positive response to intravenously or orally administered antiepileptic drugs, e.g., phenytoin or valproic acid. Some (no more than 10%) of the patients also have epileptic seizures of the grand mal type, some exhibit signs and symptoms of multiple sclerosis.

38.5 Psychogenic Unilateral Fits

Finally, a psychogenic origin of unilateral fits is not infrequent, and in this case the fits are in most instances motor, not sensory, in nature. The diagnosis rests on the patient's personal observation, which does not reveal tonic-clonic or choreoathetotic movements unless he has had the opportunity to observe these in other persons. Rather, the movements may have expressive features, or may inhibit any use of the limb, e.g., by simultaneous innervation of the flexor and extensor muscles. One should not expect the patient to conform to the stereotype of the "hysterical personality", nor can one expect to learn of personal tensions without knowing the patient quite well. EEG is normal during these seizures.

39 Vertigo

Vertigo may be paroxysmal or of long duration. In both cases it is experienced by many patients as an alarming event or condition. As a result, description of vertigo is frequently not very clear, and history taking requires both sound knowledge of the clinical varieties and a good deal of patience. We distinguish directional vertigo from unsystematic dizziness. Directional, mostly rotating vertigo must be attributed to functional disturbance of one labyrinth, because only there are the directions in space represented separately. Unsystematic dizziness results from functional disturbance in higher levels of the vestibular system, where specific directional information is integrated.

39.1 Benign Paroxysmal Positional Vertigo

By far the most frequent type is benign paroxysmal positional vertigo. Usually, the patient reports apparent rotation of his surroundings and unsteadiness of body posture, accompanied by a feeling of anxiety and, sometimes, nausea. Acoustic symptoms such as tinnitus are not present. The single attack lasts only a few seconds, but it may recur in an unpredictable fashion. It takes some questioning to find out that vertigo is regularly precipitated by assuming a certain position of the head, such as bending down to tie shoelaces or perform some other task, lying down, or turning around in bed. Some patients have their attacks when they change their sleeping position. It is always one and the same position that precipitates the attack. Many patients are not aware of this, yet they instinctively avoid assuming the critical position.

As soon as the diagnosis is suspected one should proceed to place the patient in various positions, preferably observing him for nystagmus with the help of Frenzel's glasses. It is mandatory that the patient does not lie down before the examination starts, but rather awaits the doctor sitting on the examination couch. The reason is that positional vertigo tends to habituate very fast, so that it may be weaker the second time the critical position is assumed, and absent the third time. The attack begins with a latency of some seconds. During an attack there is usually rotating nystagmus beating toward the undermost ear. The vertigo abates after roughly a minute. The direction of nystagmus is reversed when the patient returns to the seated position. Repeat examination will demonstrate attenuation and finally absence of vertigo, which is crucial for the diagnosis and at the same time will convince the patient of the rationale for therapy (see below).

Except for positional nystagmus the neurologic status is normal, as are caloric responses. Ancillary examinations are not necessary. This type of vertigo is benign; it is not a premonitory symptom of any disease of the nervous system, especially not of acoustic neuroma or of posterior fossa tumor. Drug therapy is of little help. The only effective therapy is positional exercise, which presumably disseminates the detritus detached from the otoliths either spontaneously or after head trauma (so-called cupulolithiasis). The exercise is done by having the patient assume the precipitating position several times every 3 hours until vertigo subsides.

39.2 "Vestibular Neuronitis"

Vertigo of abrupt onset, associated with nausea and directional nystagmus, but not with tinnitus or other cochlear symptoms, is denoted by the traditional term vestibular neuronitis. Movements of the head aggravate the vertigo, but it is also present at rest. Intensity may fluctuate. Caloric tests are abnormal on one or both sides. In rare cases there are signs of brain stem dysfunction or unspecific bilateral abnormality in the EEG. In these cases mild brain stem encephalitis is suspected. Neurologic findings are otherwise normal. The condition is felt to be of infective origin; it sometimes has a limited epidemic spread ("epidemic vertigo"). Prognosis is good.

39.3 Menière's Disease

A chronic condition, Menière's disease is characterized by regular attacks of mostly rotating vertigo and nystagmus with nausea and vomiting, accompanied by tinnitus and frequently also by signs and symptoms of the autonomic nervous system, such as sweating, diarrhea, and alteration of cardiac frequency and of blood pressure. Many patients are not able to maintain the erect position during the attack, preferring to lie down on one side, which indicates the nonaffected ear. The single attack is not triggered by a recognizable event or position. It lasts for hours, in rare cases for several days, and is usually followed by some days of uncharacteristic dizziness and malaise. Usually there has been unilateral hearing loss and tinnitus for months or years before the first attack.

Otologic examination reveals unilateral canal paresis, or at least directional preponderance and impairment of hearing. Loudness recruitment is positive, suggesting labyrinthine damage. Symptoms and signs are so characteristic that it appears superfluous to initiate the usual neuroradiological search for tumor of the cerebellopontine angle. These tumors never produce attacks of vertigo of the Menière type.

39.4 Concussion of the Labyrinth

Vertigo with vomiting or dizziness following cranial trauma usually suggests benign concussion of the labyrinth. The symptoms last several days or weeks and gradually subside. There are no cochlear symptoms. If there are (loud unilateral tinnitus and/or hearing loss), and if vertigo and nausea are particularly intense, fracture of the petrous bone should be suspected. Radiological and ear, nose, and throat (ENT) examination are urgent, because immediate surgical therapy might be indicated.

39.5 Herpes Zoster Oticus

Although apparently easy, the diagnosis of herpes zoster oticus contains some pitfalls. The presenting symptoms may be rotatory vertigo with nausea and tinnitus. Many patients feel pain in the ear, the lateral face, or the nuchal region, but this symptom is ambiguous. After 2 or 3 days, the typical vesicles appear. These may be hidden deep in the external ear or on the tympanic membrane, and thereby escape detection if not deliberately searched for. In this case, paralysis of other cranial nerves may divert diagnostic attention to the group of conditions discussed in Chap. 21. There may be paralysis of the facial, trigeminal, abducent, vagal, and hypoglossal nerves. Some patients have singultus, which arouses the suspicion of brain tumor, but in this setting it indicates hyperexcitability of the complex of the vagal nucleus. CSF shows increased cell count and protein level.

Diagnosis rests on demonstration of the vesicles. Serological tests are not of immediate help, because a positive result can be expected only after 2–3 days.

39.6 Intoxication

Unsystematic dizziness is one of the features of functional disturbance of the brain stem. The most frequent cause of brain stem disorder today is chronic intoxication. The most commonly taken drugs acting on the brain stem are benzodiazepines, barbiturates, and antiepileptics, the latter normally unwittingly taken in overdose. As a rule, dizziness is accompanied by nystagmus on sideward gaze, slightly slurred speech, and a mild decrease in reactivity. EEG and toxicologic findings confirm the diagnosis (see also Chap. 10).

39.7 Other Brain Stem Disease

Other diseases of the brain stem that frequently cause dizziness are multiple sclerosis and basilar artery insufficiency. The latter diagnosis has been in use for nearly 2 decades in a somewhat inflationary way. It should be made with caution and only on the basis of strong signs and symptoms suggestive of vascular disease of the hindbrain circulation. Definitely, degenerative disease of the cervical vertebrae does not interfere with flow in the vertebral arteries to an extent that dizziness or any other symptom ensues. This has been convincingly demonstrated by CW ultrasound studies. Even when the head was turned excessively to one side so that flow in the ipsilateral vertebral artery was reduced at the level of the occipitocervical junction, there was compensatory increase of flow in the contralateral artery, and the elderly subjects did not experience vertigo or any other unpleasant sensation.

39.8 Tumor of the Cerebellopontine Angle

One of the diagnoses that occur to most doctors if a patient complains of vertigo is tumor of the cerebellopontine angle. However, directional vertigo is very rare, although the tumors arise from or compress the eighth nerve. Even unsystematic dizziness is not a prominent symptom, although large tumors compress the brain stem. On the contrary, the contrast between the coarse nystagmus as described in Chap. 21 and the paucity of subjective symptoms is striking.

39.9 Infarction or Tumor of the Cerebellum

The situation is quite different in cerebellar infarction and tumor. Here, vertigo and ataxia are among the leading symptoms. Vertigo is usually not rotatory, but directed to one side or backward, and is thus clearly differentiated from the dizziness in disease of the brain stem and of the cerebral hemispheres.

Acute or rapidly progressive onset suggests vascular etiology. In this case, further symptoms to be expected are: unilateral locomotor or trunk ataxia, lesions of the lower cranial nerves, and sensory disturbance in one half of the body or in "crossed distribution" on one side of the face and the opposite side of the body. There may be Horner's syndrome.

In cerebellar tumor, there is occipital headache aggravated by coughing or by rising from a supine to a sitting position, nausea, and frequently papilledema. Incidentally, large infarctions may compress the fourth ventricle and brain stem, and may even cause obstructive hydrocephalus. Doppler sonography is very helpful in detecting stenosis or occlusion in large vessels of the hindbrain circulation. Differentiation is made by neuroimaging techniques.

39.10 Hemispheric Tumor

Patients with hemispheric tumor frequently describe "dizziness," but they are never very specific about it. It is true that in the parietal lobe there is an area of multisensory integration that also receives vestibular input. In my experience, however, complaint of dizziness in patients with brain tumor mainly refers to attenuation of vigilance, i.e., reactivity, and a general feeling of being ill.

By the same token, the often-cited vertiginous epileptic aura is an extremely rare symptom.

39.11 Presbyvertigo in Degenerative Vertebral Disease

"Presbyvertigo" is a new term proposed for dizziness upon retroflexion of the head in elderly persons. The mechanism certainly is not vascular (see Sect. 39.7). It is assumed that degenerative alteration of the small intravertebral joints leads to excessive discharge of proprioceptive afferent impulses. This results in a mismatch in the elaboration of input from various sensory modalities, which, again, may cause dizziness.

39.12 Psychogenic Vertigo

One should not lose sight of the fact that complaint of dizziness may just be the expression of *psychic insecurity* rather than physical unsteadiness. The diagnoses range from depressive illness to personality problems. They cannot be discussed here in detail.

40 Weakness Upon Exercise

40.1 Myasthenia Gravis

It is well known that weakness upon exercise is the basic complaint of patients suffering from myasthenia gravis. In the beginning of the disease there is no weakness at all in the morning, after a night's rest, but the patients notice a decrease in muscular strength during activities of various kinds. It depends on the affection of the muscles or groups of muscles which these activities – ranging from reading, speaking, and similar activities to walking or all kinds of manual work (e.g., typing or pressing a lever in industrial work) – require. Periods of rest restore strength at least partially, and weakness is greatest in the evening.

Suspicion of myasthenia should prompt a simple capacity test, which requires the patient to perform as often as 30–40 times those movements that are reported to be impaired. Examples are: opening and closing the eyes forcefully, counting, lifting the head in a supine position, and pressing a dynamometer. If there is a decrease in force (or voice), pharmacologic tests are warranted. Injection of inhibitors of cholinesterase (e.g., neostigmine) will restore strength with a latency of between 30 s and 2 min for periods of between several minutes and half an hour. The longer the period of restoration, the more likely it is that this is an unusual case which should be explored further by a specialist. One should be ready to give an additional injection of atropine, because some patients experience strong cholinergic side effects of the drug. In order to rule out psychogenic weakness, we first give an injection of saline.

Electric stimulation of a peripheral nerve leads to a decrement of action potentials in the respective muscles that is likewise reversed by cholinesterase inhibitors or substances acting on the postsynaptic membrane (edrophonium hydrochloride).

Once the diagnosis is made, further examinations are necessary. The patient should be examined for serum antibodies against acetylcholine receptors and skeletal muscles, and for thymoma or persistence of the thymus gland. Some hyperthyroid patients develop myasthenic weakness.

155

40.2 Eaton Lambert Syndrome

A paraneoplastic disease that has the abnormal fatigability in common with myasthenia, Eaton Lambert syndrome, also has nevertheless distinctive features that permit differentiation. Weakness does not begin in the extraocular or facial muscles, and, in fact, these quite often remain spared. Most affected are the muscles of the shoulder or pelvic girdle. While the patients complain of weakness upon exercise, examination reveals that on repeated innervation of affected muscles strength will increase for the first contractions and decrease only after exercise of a minute or longer. This corresponds to the characteristic findings in stimulation electromyography, where, again, the amplitude of action potentials shows first increment, then decrement. Pharmacologic tests as described in Sect. 40.1 have little, if any, effect. The syndrome is much more frequent in men, and the underlying malignancy is oat cell carcinoma of the lung in 70% of cases.

40.3 Paroxysmal Hypokalemic Paralysis

A disturbance in potassium metabolism, affecting the musculature, causes paroxysmal hypokalemic paralysis. The leading symptom is periodic paralysis of the trunk and limbs, which lasts for hours. The facial muscles and the diaphragm, as a rule, are spared. The majority of attacks occur in the night with no recognizable cause. Physical exertion however, may provoke attacks, as may meals that are rich in carbohydrates.

During the attack, the serum level of potassium drops dramatically, sometimes as low as 2 or 1.7 mval/l, and the electromyogram may be silent, i.e., show no spontaneous or action potentials. In milder attacks, amplitudes are low and duration is shortened.

In case of doubt, attacks may be provoked for diagnostic purposes by oral administration of a high dose of glucose plus 20 units of insulin s.c.

40.4 Intermittent Claudication of the Cauda Equina

Transient weakness in the legs occurs in some patients, usually of advanced age, as soon as they stand erect. Weakness is greatly aggravated by walking, sometimes to such a degree that the patient has to sit down, or he will drop to the floor. Each time the symptoms start with pain in the calves, followed by numbness in the feet that may ascend to the upper legs. Peripheral pulses remain normal, which helps to distinguish the condition from claudication of peripheral vascular origin. In contrast, proprioceptive reflexes may be attenuated, at first only during the attacks of weakness, but later on they are permanently diminished or absent. Likewise, in the initial stage nerve conduction study may in the beginning show slowing of conduction during the attack. Later on nerve conduction study and EMG findings indicate chronic damage to the cauda equina.

Radiography, in particular spinal neuroimaging, shows a narrow spinal channel. Usually, the cause is a combination of severe degenerative vertebral disease with arthrotic appositions to the intervertebral joints and some degree of protrusion of one or more intervertebral discs. One should be careful, however, not to confound the radiographic findings with the clinical picture: not in every case of narrowing of the spinal channel are there the typical symptoms and signs which alone should prompt myelographic examination. This examination should be done in both lordotic and kyphotic curvature of the spine. The relevant finding is interruption of the passage of contrast medium, at least in lordosis. The mechanism is certainly complex, and involves both direct pressure on the roots of the cauda equina and interference with blood flow in the radicular arteries. Therapy is surgical.

41 Wrist Drop

41.1 How to Differentiate Peripheral and Central Wrist Drop

Wrist drop is a sign equally as treacherous as footdrop (see Chap.
16). Again, it has first to be established whether the weakness of elevation is peripheral or central. A simple and effective way of distinguishing between the two is to ask the patient to grasp the doctor's hand
firmly. In this movement, there is normally simultaneous contraction
of the long extensor and flexor muscles of the forearm, in order to
keep the wrist fixed in the stretched position which is required to permit
a strong flexion of the fingers.

In the case of *radial nerve palsy* the wrist drop becomes even more
pronounced, i.e., maximal flexion of the hand results upon the maneuver. In the case of *central paresis*, there will be slight elevation of
the hand and some mass action on the neighboring joints, such as
flexion at the elbow. Also, wrist drop due to *radial nerve palsy* is accompanied by weakness of finger extension. The extensor digitorum longus
muscle acts on the carpometacarpal joint in each of fingers 2–5. Hence,
by placing his index finger under the first phalanx of these fingers,
the doctor supports this function, and compensates for radial nerve
dysfunction, and stretching of the fingers in the interphalangeal joints
will be possible because this is a function supplied by the ulnar nerve.

Eliciting the two reflexes where the radial nerve is involved may
be equally helpful. If the lesion affects the radial nerve high on the
upper arm, the triceps reflex and the radial stretch reflex will both
be diminished or absent. If the lesion is located immediately above
the elbow, the triceps reflex may be normal and only the radial stretch
reflex diminished.

There is one location of damage to the radial nerve which leaves
both reflexes unaffected. This is in the forearm, directly below the
elbow joint, within the supinator muscle. But in this case the extensor
carpi radialis muscle will be spared, with the result that there is only
incomplete wrist drop which is due to weakness of the extensor carpi
ulnaris muscle.

In central weakness, reflexes are, of course, brisker on the affected side.

Finally, testing cutaneous sensory functions yields characteristic findings. The area of supply of the radial nerve is on the dorsal aspect of the thumb and index fingers, and on the back of the hand immediately adjacent to these. Only in the case of supinator longus syndrome is there no sensory deficit, but this condition is recognized by its motor symptoms, as indicated above.

Central wrist drop either leaves cutaneous sensibility unaffected or the entire hand numb.

It goes without saying that measurement of nerve conduction velocity in most cases supplies an answer to the question: is the lesion peripheral or central, and if peripheral, where exactly is it located? The scope of this book, however, is to make the examiner as independent as possible of ancillary examinations.

41.2 Peripheral: Radial Nerve Lesion

When the peripheral origin has been established, the next problem is to establish whether the patient has an isolated lesion of the radial nerve, or whether the "radial nerve palsy" is part of widespread disease of the peripheral nervous system, in other words, of polyneuropathy.

Except in the case of unambiguous situations like wrist drop following fracture of the humerus or surgical therapy, including plaster cast, it is advisable to examine the functions of the other peripheral nerves of the four limbs. The reason is that a lesion of the radial nerve is not infrequently promoted by a preexisting polyneuropathy, which had been "silent" up to the occurrence of wrist drop. The best-known example is lead polyneuropathy. Radial nerve weakness may also be the first sign of polyarteritis nodosa, which eventually affects the vasa nervorum of all peripheral nerves. Also, diabetic metabolic derangement brings about a predisposition to compression neuropathy.

Compression neuropathy is the most frequent cause of isolated peripheral wrist drop. The most popular example is the "Saturday night palsy," caused by pressure of the upper arm against the back of a park bench when the person is in such a state of drunkenness that the warning pinprick sensations which invariably precede any compression paralysis are not perceived. The romantic names "bridegroom palsy," or in French "paralysie des amants," refer to the effect of pressure exerted by the head of the sleeping partner on the abducted upper arm.

41.3 Central: Lacunar Stroke or Occlusion of Peripheral Branch of Middle Cerebral Artery

Central wrist drop is almost exclusively of vascular etiology. It is due to occlusion of a small vessel mostly in the peripheral, i.e., subcortical, distribution of branches of the middle cerebral artery. The ensuing small lesions are called lacunes, and the type of stroke, lacunar stroke. It is due to hypertensive arteriopathy, and neuroimaging frequently permits the recognition of a typical arteriopathic pattern, by showing either other lacunes that are asymptomatic at that point in time, or diffuse areas of hypodensity in the white matter of the hemispheres and/or surrounding the anterior and posterior horn of the lateral ventricles. This is characteristic of Binswanger's subcortical arteriosclerotic encephalopathy.

Subject Index

Main entrances in **boldface**

166

K. Poeck   Diagnostic Decisions in Neurology

Erratum

Page 27, 2nd paragraph, 4th line

- Jackson's famous dictum that the brain (i.e., the cortex) does not know
of muscles, it knows only of movements. One would not call a wristdrop
resulting from stroke a central paralysis of the radial nerve, or a foot-

Page 39, Section 10.4, 11th line

- clinical means alone. In both instances there may be hydrocephalus
due to compression of the fourth ventricle. Recognition of the space-
occupying nature of the lesion is vital, because tumors and hem-

Page 40, Section 10.6 last line

- angiography. A lumbar tap may threaten the patient's life, because
lowering of spinal CSF pressure relative to intracranial CSF pressure
may lead to herniation of the cerebellum into the foramen magnum.

Springer-Verlag Berlin Heidelberg New York Tokyo